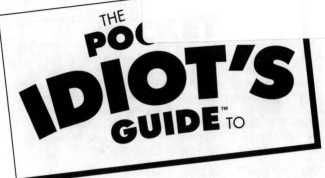

THE

POCKET IDIOT'S GUIDE™ TO

A Good Night's Sleep

by Dr. Martin Moore-Ede and Suzanne LeVert

alpha books

A Division of Macmillan General Reference
A Pearson Education Macmillan Company
1633 Broadway, New York, NY 10019-6785

Macmillan Publishing books may be purchased for business or sales promotional use. For information please write: Special Markets Department, Macmillan Publishing USA, 1633 Broadway, New York, NY 10019.

International Standard Book Number: 0-02-863380-6
Library of Congress Catalog Card Number: 99-62693

01   00   99   8   7   6   5   4   3   2   1

Interpretation of the printing code: the rightmost number of the first series of numbers is the year of the book's printing; the rightmost number of the second series of numbers is the number of the book's printing. For example, a printing code of 99-1 shows that the first printing occurred in 1999.

Printed in the United States of America

Note: This publication contains the opinions and ideas of its authors. It is intended to provide helpful and informative material on the subject matter covered. It is sold with the understanding that the authors and publisher are not engaged in rendering professional services in the book. If the reader requires personal assistance or advice, a competent professional should be consulted.

Book Producer
Amaranth

Alpha Development Team

Publisher
Kathy Nebenhaus

Editorial Director
Gary M. Krebs

Managing Editor
Bob Shuman

Marketing Brand Manager
Felice Primeau

Acquisitions Editor
Jessica Faust

Development Editors
Phil Kitchel
Amy Zavatto

Assistant Editor
Georgette Blau

Production Team

Development Editor
Lee Ann Chearney/Amaranth

Production Editor
Michael Thomas

Copy Editor
Heather Gregory

Cover Designer
Mike Freeland

Photo Editor
Richard H. Fox

Illustrator
Jody P. Schaeffer

Book Designers
Scott Cook and Amy Adams of DesignLab

Indexer
Tonya Heard

Layout/Proofreading
Melissa Auciello-Brogan
Julie Trippetti

Contents

Introduction

Do you feel like an idiot because you can't get to sleep at night or because you drag yourself through the day feeling only half awake? Well, don't despair. We've written this book just for you and the millions of other sleep-deprived Americans who just can't seem to get the sleep they need to feel alive and well every day. Indeed, sleep is one of the most precious yet underrated commodities of the day. In this book, you'll learn all about your own unique "sleep personality," which determines your optimum sleep patterns, as well as how to track down specific sleep problems that could be keeping you up at night. Chock full of easy-to-follow practical tips, *The Pocket Idiot's Guide ™ to a Good Night's Sleep* will help you get all the zzzz's you need!

Extras

In addition to helpful advice and information, this book provides sidebars throughout the text to explain unfamiliar terms, warn you against dangerous habits or situations, and give you helpful tips. Look for these easy-to-recognize signposts:

Words to Sleep By

The vocabulary of sleep and sleep medicine.

Rest Easy

Expert advice on improving your chances of getting a good night's sleep.

Set Your Alarm!

Warnings about potentially harmful habits that interfere with sleep.

Trademarks

All terms mentioned in this book that are known to be or are suspected of being trademarks or service marks have been appropriately capitalized. Alpha books and Macmillan General Reference cannot attest to the accuracy of this information. Use of a term in this book should not be regarded as affecting the validity of any trademark or service mark.

The Story of Sleep

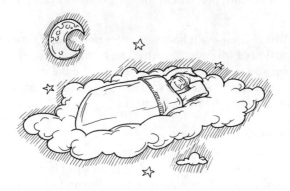

In This Chapter

➤ The need for sleep

➤ Are you sleep deprived?

➤ The enemies of sleep

It seems like it should be the easiest thing in the world, doesn't it? Just lie back, close your eyes, and drift off into the blissful oblivion called sleep. Then, about eight hours later, you wake up feeling refreshed and renewed, ready to meet the challenge of staying awake and alert for the next sixteen hours. That's the way it *should* work, right? Unfortunately, sleep isn't always that simple, nor is maintaining this standard sleep/wake schedule.

If you spend your nights tossing and turning instead of snoozing away, or if the demands of modern life interfere with your normal sleep schedule, you're far from alone. Lack of sleep is now a widespread modern problem: According to the National Sleep Foundation, nearly half of all Americans suffer from insomnia and other sleep-related disorders, and a recent Gallup survey reports that 56 percent of the adult population experience problems with daytime drowsiness. Indeed, lack of sleep has become a major health problem in the United States and around the world.

In this chapter, we'll help you better understand your biological need for sleep and what can happen to your body when you go without it. We'll also outline the most common enemies of sleep, as well as help you determine if you're among the sleep deprived.

Fatigue Kills

Since you're reading this book, chances are you've spent a few sleepless nights yourself and know just how awful a night or two of poor sleep or no sleep can feel. From grouchiness to nausea to an inability to concentrate, the symptoms of *sleep deprivation* are uncomfortable and debilitating—and the side effects not only can interfere with your ability to enjoy a productive day, but actually can be deadly.

Words to Sleep By

Sleep deprivation is a term used to describe the state you're in when you do not obtain enough sleep to satisfy your body's needs.

Just take a look at these shocking facts about sleep deprivation in the United States today:

> ➤ More than 30 percent of American drivers admit to having fallen asleep at the wheel at least once in

their lifetime, and the National Sleep Foundation estimates that at least 100,000 accidents and 1,500 fatalities per year are due to drivers falling asleep at the wheel.

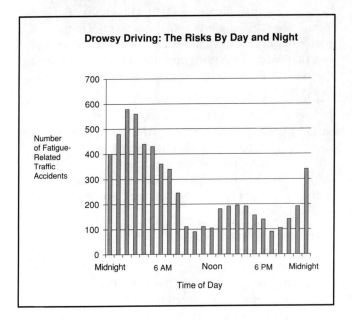

Drowsy Driving: The Risks By Day and Night

Number of Fatigue-Related Traffic Accidents

This graph shows that, by far, most drowsy driver accidents take place during the wee hours of the morning—between midnight and 6 a.m—with another increase in mid-afternoon.

After Mitler MM et al, Sleep 11: 100-109, 1988 with permission.

➤ The National Transportation Safety Board reported that "Fatigue is the No. 1 factor that detrimentally impacts the ability of pilots."

➤ Thirty percent of high school and college students fall asleep in class at least once a week.

➤ The direct costs of human fatigue to the American economy are about $70 billion per year—and world-wide, the figure may be as high as $300 billion.

Pretty big numbers, no? And all blamed on the lack of sleep, an essential physiological function most of us neglect. Indeed, sleep is probably the most underrated source of health and vitality available to the human race, one that we consistently ignore and discount. The consequences are not just economic, but very personal as well.

No doubt you already know how much a lack of sleep affects your ability to function. If you're running a power saw or performing a heart transplant when you're sleepy, the consequences can be fatal. But even if you're not involved in a potentially dangerous activity, sleep deprivation can be uncomfortable and upsetting. In addition to itchy eyes, which is the most universal symptom, several other problems arise:

➤ **Mood changes**. Irritability, depression, and anxiety are the three most common mood disturbances caused by lack of sleep. But we don't need to tell you that, do we? When you haven't satisfied your sleep needs, you're grouchy or miserable or twitchy (or maybe all three), aren't you? You also may feel overwhelmed and anxious facing even small challenges on too little sleep.

➤ **Decreased cognitive function**. Ever try to concentrate when you're sleep deprived, especially on something boring like balancing your checkbook or performing another routine task? If you're even a little sleep deprived, such tasks make you sleepier yet, don't they? Ready to nod off? (In fact, you may well be nodding off: Many people who are sleep deprived suffer "microsleeps," brief episodes of sleep lasting only a few seconds.) Mistakes get made, big time, by the sleep deprived, which can get mighty dangerous if your job is tracking planes across busy corridors in the sky as an air-traffic controller or watching children play near the deep end of the pool.

➤ **Decreased motor skills**. Same goes here. Hand-eye coordination just isn't the same when you don't get enough sleep. And neither are your reflexes—the semi-automatic moves you make under certain circumstances, like braking or swerving when you see a puppy run out in front of your car, slow down when you're sleep-deprived.

➤ **Weight gain**. Yup. Not sleeping is definitely a risk factor when it comes to gaining weight. Think about it: What do you reach for when you're tired? A candy bar, a soft drink, a doughnut—any quick, high-carbohydrate, high-sugar food to give you a boost when you're dragging. Unfortunately, not only will this approach backfire and leave you feeling more tired than ever, but if your sleep problem is chronic, you'll start gaining weight as those snacks pile up.

➤ **Impaired immune system**. It isn't your imagination: You really do run a greater risk of getting a cold or other infection when you lack sleep. We now know that lack of sleep undermines your immune system's ability to fight off foreign intruders like viruses and bacteria.

As you can see, you need to sleep well on a regular basis in order to maintain your health and function efficiently and safely in your daily life. But why, exactly, is that true? What *is* sleep, anyway?

The Art of Sleep

To be able to sleep, and sleep well, isn't as easy as it sounds. In fact, sleep is a downright complex behavior, involving a wide range of physiological activities. You fall asleep and then wake up as your body temperature falls and rises in a distinct pattern. Hormones secreted by various endocrine glands help set up the internal environment for periods of sleep and wakefulness, working with your brain in a delicate and intricate dance throughout the day and night.

The key to this process is the internal body clock, which each of us inherits from our parents along with our other unique attributes. Your body has a rhythm all its own, and left to its own devices would "choose" to sleep a specific amount of time at certain times of the day. Understanding your own personal rhythm, which may differ from other people's, and learning to adapt it to a different schedule—occasionally or on an on-going basis—without becoming sleep deprived is essential to good health and a productive life.

Set Your Alarm!

If you have trouble sleeping and can't figure out why, try looking no further than the other side of your bed. Is your partner's tossing and turning, snoring and fidgeting, or chronic blanket snatching keeping you awake? If so, it may be time for one of you to sleep in the guest room until the problem is resolved.

The amount of stress in your life and your ability to cope with it, your diet, and your exercise habits also have a definite impact on how much and how well you sleep. Needless to say, it's often difficult to fall asleep when you're tense with worry and anxiety, or when too much caffeine stimulates the brain just when you want it to slow down. Although getting some exercise doesn't automatically mean a good night's sleep, people who exercise on a regular basis tend to suffer from less depression and anxiety, conditions that often disrupt sleep. Exercisers also tend not to be overweight, a risk factor for snoring and a breathing disorder called Obstructive Sleep Apnea, two other enemies of sleep.

In this book, we'll show you what you need to change in your life and environment to prepare your body and mind for sleep every night. First, let's figure out *why* you need to sleep.

Everybody Needs Sleep!

Why is sleep so important? What function does it serve to the human body and mind? Unfortunately, no one really knows the precise answers to these questions. There are, however, many different theories:

> ➤ **Rest.** It seems pretty obvious that one reason we sleep—perhaps the main reason—is that sleep helps to "recharge" our physical and psychological batteries. At the same time, however, we know that certain parts of the brain work harder during sleep than during wakefulness. So providing us with rest is not the whole sleep story. Indeed, feeling fatigued after a hard day's work is only one of the reasons we fall asleep; automatic changes in body temperature and hormone levels have a lot to do with it, too.

> ➤ **Growth and repair.** Sleep appears to help body cells grow and regenerate. During deep sleep in the early part of the night, the endocrine system secretes human growth hormone (HGH), a body chemical that stimulates the growth of muscle and organ tissues. During adulthood, the hormone acts to trigger the repair of these tissues.

➤ **Energy conservation**. When you're awake, your body burns a great deal of oxygen and food to provide energy for daily physical and mental activities. Called "catabolism," this process burns up your energy reserves. During sleep, your body is more anabolic, meaning it conserves energy. For instance, when you're asleep, both your body temperature and your metabolism (the rate at which you burn energy) falls. In essence, sleep gives the body a break from its daily physiological activities.

➤ **Memory consolidation and discharge of emotions**. Some researchers believe that sleep helps reinforce memories, whereas dreaming—a natural part of the sleep process—helps sort and purge deep-seated emotional issues.

➤ **Safety**. In many mammals, sleep offers respite from food chain activity. In other words, a mouse asleep in its burrow is unlikely to attract the attention of a prowling, hungry cat. Even humans are safer, for the most part, when they're asleep in their own beds than when they're awake and crossing the street against the light or even going up and down the stairs at home.

Now that you know why you need to sleep, it's time to figure why it's so hard for you to do just that.

Why It's *So* Hard Sometimes

Most Americans can find their enemies in their own lifestyles. They're too busy, stressed, underexercised, and overweight to sleep well. In other cases, medical sleep disorders interfere with proper sleep. Here's a quick rundown of the most common enemies:

➤ **Insomnia**. Insomnia is a general term for a variety of problems having to do with getting and staying asleep. Literally, the word *insomnia* means "no sleep" during a 24-hour period, but most people who suffer with insomnia get at least some sleep. Insomnia can be transient (lasting only a night or two on an occasional basis), short-term (lasting from three nights to three weeks), or chronic (long-lasting and intransigent). In some cases, insomnia can be traced to a medical problem; in others, a lifestyle issue; and in still others, no cause can be found.

➤ **Disruption of sleep patterns.** Sometimes for no known reason, sometimes because of shift work or travel across time zones, your sleep patterns become disrupted. You fall asleep and wake up too early or too late to keep company with the world around you. Such problems usually require the help of a sleep specialist to solve. In Chapters 10, 11, and 12, we discuss such disturbances in more depth.

➤ **Snoring and sleep apnea** (yours or your partner's). Author Anthony Burgess once wrote, "Laugh and the world laughs with you; snore and you snore alone." Simple snoring not only interferes with your partner's sleep, but also often disrupts your ability to sleep deeply yourself. Its close relative Obstructive Sleep Apnea is even more serious. Sleep apnea causes breathing to stop from 10 seconds up to a minute at a time, after which you wake up for a few seconds, often gasping for breath, and then fall back asleep—sometimes without ever realizing you've been disturbed. We discuss snoring and sleep apnea, and some solutions to them, in Chapter 9.

➤ **Parasomnias** (yours or your partner's). Walking and talking after midnight can be sexy, sweet pastimes—as long as you're not actually sound asleep while you're doing them. Teeth-grinding and night terrors (startling, upsetting, partial or total awakenings from deep sleep) are other parasomnias. Other disturbing disorders include Restless Leg Syndrome, which is characterized by discomfort in the legs relieved by movement, and Periodic Limb Movements in Sleep, characterized by repetitive leg movements or jerks. Clearly, both can wreak havoc on sleep for anyone who happens to be in the bed. We explain these problems in more depth in Chapter 10.

➤ **Medical illness.** Infections, allergies, pain, indigestion, and many other medical conditions have sleep problems as side effects. In addition, the drugs you take to treat these and other illnesses may also cause insomnia.

Set Your Alarm!

A sleep problem is a common symptom of depression, anxiety, and a wide variety of physical ailments including diabetes, asthma, and arthritis. That's why it's important to see your doctor to rule out other causes for your sleep difficulties or chronic fatigue. You may need treatment for the underlying illness as well as for your difficulties with sleep.

➤ **Emotional disturbances.** A recent divorce, the death of a loved one, work pressures, a bout of the blues: Any of these emotional difficulties—commonly lumped together under the heading of "stress"—can interfere with your ability to get to sleep and stay asleep. The solutions we discuss later can help someone with a temporary emotional upset get better sleep.

How Much Is Enough?

Ah, that perennial question that too often has led to a pat response: What's enough? Eight hours. It's true that the average adult seems to exist on eight hours, or, more technically, about seven and a half hours of sleep. That's not to say, however, that seven and a half hours is the standard amount of sleep that you as an individual need or even desire. Some sleep studies show that, given their druthers, many people would choose to sleep about eight to nine hours on a regular basis. The fact that most of us consistently get less than that shows just how widespread sleep deprivation has come to be.

That said, sleep requirements and preferences are highly individual things. They vary from person to person, under different circumstances, and at different times of life. Generally speaking, though, there are at least four categories of sleep behavior:

➤ **Long sleepers vs. short sleepers.** Some people need nine or ten hours of sleep in order to feel well, while others thrive on just five or six.

➤ **Rigid sleepers vs. flexible sleepers.** Some people wake up at the same time every morning no matter what time they go to bed, even if they've slept only a few hours. Others can easily adjust their sleep patterns to accommodate changes in their normal social or work schedules.

➤ **Larks vs. owls.** No doubt you've heard of this category already: The morning people—those who do their best work at the crack of dawn—and the night people—those who don't really come alive until evening.

➤ **Nappers vs. non-nappers.** Some people are able to make up for lost sleep time by taking a nap, whereas others simply have to exist through the day until their next nocturnal sleep period. Dedicated nappers find that a daily nap becomes an essential part of their sleep/wake pattern, and that they don't function as well on days when they miss that afternoon snooze.

In Chapter 3, you'll discover what your "Sleep Personality" is, and how it affects your ability to get enough regular sleep. You'll also learn how to keep a "Sleep Log" so that you'll know exactly how much sleep you get and how you feel at various times during the day. We'll also help you to understand how your work, family, and social life affect your sleep patterns and how to make the most out of the schedule you have today.

Rest Easy

Don't assume you have a sleep problem if you sleep more or less than the average 7½ hours a night. If you wake up feeling refreshed and alert and function well during the day, on a regular basis, chances are you're getting just the right amount of sleep for you.

Is it possible to exist on four, five, or six hours of sleep a night? Absolutely. As long as you wake up feeling rested, and remain alert throughout the day, you'll be just fine. Are you ill if you need to sleep nine or ten hours a day? Not at all. Consider this: We estimate that the average person 100 years ago, before the electric light bulb ruled the night, slept about eight to nine hours daily. Today, the average person sleeps just seven and a half hours a night—and millions complain of feeling chronically tired and out of sorts.

Do you believe that you sleep enough and feel rested when you wake up? Or is it possible that you are among the millions of sleep-deprived walking the streets of America today? The following quiz will help you determine your sleep status.

Are You Getting Enough Sleep?

1. I wish I had more energy.
   Yes ___ No ___

2. I frequently have a headache in the morning.
   Yes ___ No ___

3. I often have to struggle during the day to remain alert.
   Yes ___ No ___

4. I often have trouble concentrating.
   Yes ___ No ___

5. I seem to tire easily when performing physical tasks.
   Yes ___ No ___

6. I seem to be particularly susceptible to colds and other infections.
   Yes ___ No ___

7. I often feel like I'm going to fall asleep while driving.
   Yes ___ No ___

8. I often feel like I'm in a daze.
   Yes ___ No ___

9. My friends and family say that I tend to be often grumpy and irritable.
   Yes ___ No ___

10. I worry about things and have trouble relaxing.
    Yes ___ No ___

If you've answered more than three or four of these questions with a yes, you may be able to trace your difficulty to a sleep problem. At the same time—and we'll say this more than once in this book—these same behaviors and symptoms may indicate a physical or psychological problem that requires treatment or advice from a medical doctor. If you're having chronic sleep problems, you should make an appointment with your doctor for a check-up to rule out other causes.

Finding the Secret to Sleep

The good news is that for almost every common sleep problem, there is a solution. Some solutions involve making lifestyle changes, like cutting back on caffeine or changing your diet. Severe cases of sleep apnea and disturbances of the body clock may require more intensive treatment.

That's not to say that every case of insomnia is easily fixable—some can be maddeningly stubborn and the underlying cause of the problem difficult to identify. But with patience, effort, and a little trial and error, sleep may cease to be so tantalizingly out of reach.

Read on, and we'll help you figure out what's keeping you up at night and show you ways to improve the quality of your sleep. By doing so, you're sure to feel more vital, alert, and alive than ever.

Chapter 2

The Rhythms of Sleep

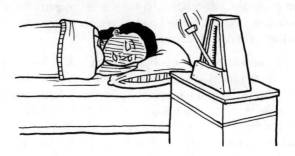

In This Chapter

➤ Understanding the internal clock

➤ Your personal rhythms

➤ The cycles of sleep

Choices: You've got a lot of them to make every day, don't you? What time to get up, when to exercise, what to eat and when, how hard to work. For the most part, you have the power to choose how you live—at least within the context of the 20th century social imperatives of work and family life. Such decisions are completely yours to make, or so it seems.

You might be surprised, however, to discover how much a powerful internal mechanism known as the biological clock influences your desires and abilities. In this chapter, we'll explore the way the biological clock works and how it influences your sleep patterns.

The Clock Inside

There are only twenty-four hours in the day, right? Well,
actually, that depends on what kind of day you're talking
about. The Earth does indeed make a complete rotation
on its axis about every 24 hours and circles around the
sun every 365¼ days. Our civilization has constructed a
clock and a calendar based on this regular cycle of light/
dark and change of season.

But we now know that the human body has its own way
of keeping time that's almost—but not quite—in harmony
with this rhythm of nature and the very rigid man-made
clock we've developed to keep track of it. Your internal
clock is far more flexible than the one that ticks on your
nightstand and desktop and is far more individual. In fact,
you have a slightly different internal rhythm than does
anyone else—which may explain why your boss seems to
be at her peak of efficiency at 8 a.m., while you're still
wiping sleep dust from your eyes!

Although the differences between your internal clock and
the man-made one—and between your natural rhythms
and those of the people around you—might be small,
those differences can strongly affect how you feel mentally, emotionally, and physically.

So exactly what does your endogenous clock keep track of
and help to coordinate? Pretty much every biological activity you can think of, from your body temperature to
the hormones that course through your bloodstream to
how often your stomach contracts. In turn, these biological events profoundly influence the way you behave and
how you feel as you go about your daily routine.

"About a Day" Body Rhythms

Because many of the body's activities occur in roughly
a 24-hour cycle (and we'll talk more about how rough
this estimate is in the next section), one of the early

researchers in this area, Franz Halberg of the University of Minnesota, named them *circadian* (Latin for "about a day") rhythms. Many of your biological activities have circadian rhythms: You probably know, for instance, that the average "normal" body temperature for humans is about 98.6°F. What you might not realize is that your temperature fluctuates in a set pattern on a daily basis. Your temperature is at its low point (about 96°F) between 4 a.m. and 6 a.m., then climbs sharply during the morning hours and more gently during the afternoon. It reaches its peak of about 99°F between 7 p.m. and 8 p.m., and then begins to fall to its low point once again.

Words to Sleep By

The term **circadian** is taken from the Latin **circa,** which means "about," and **dies,** which means "day." Circadian rhythms are those biological rhythms that recur about every 24 hours.

Internal rhythms, however, continue—body temperature rises and falls in a set pattern, for instance. In addition, experiments show that the body temperature cycle and the sleep/wake cycle are normally intimately linked: We feel more alert the higher our body temperature is (within normal limits!), and our energy and ability to concentrate tend to sag the lower the temperature falls.

Another key biological rhythm when it comes to the sleep/wake cycle is the secretion of a hormone called melatonin. The pineal gland, an endocrine organ located in the brain, releases melatonin synchronized by a signal from the *suprachiasmatic nuclei (SCN)*. Melatonin and body

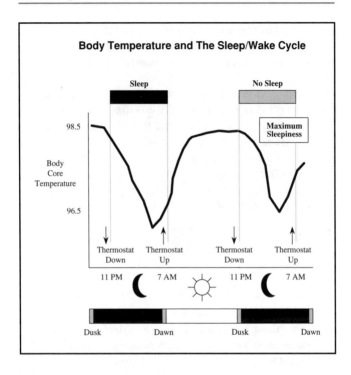

Body Temperature and The Sleep/Wake Cycle

As you can see from this graph, your body temperature— triggered by your internal body clock—starts falling as the night begins (setting the stage for sleep) and then begins to rise in the hours before dawn (helping get you ready for the day ahead). What's interesting is that this circadian rhythm of temperature rise and fall occurs whether or not you go to sleep.

temperatures rise and fall in a mirror image, together setting the stage for sleep. As our body temperature falls, the level of melatonin rises, and we begin to feel sleepy. As our temperature rises, melatonin levels fall, and we wake up. Other hormones rise and fall in a regular pattern as well: Levels of the stress hormones that ready our bodies for action, such as cortisol, start to rise as melatonin falls, stimulating us to wake up ready to face the day.

Words to Sleep By

The **suprachiasmatic nuclei**, or **SCN**, is a tiny cluster of brain cells that acts as the body's primary biological clock. It helps orchestrate the sleep/wake cycle and a host of other physiological functions.

Of course, sleep can, and does, occur at all phases of the day. But how well and how long you sleep depend a great deal on when you go to sleep. In fact, there are two "preferred" times for sleep within the 24-hour period: 1) the major one that occurs at night as the body temperature is falling (and melatonin levels are rising) and 2) one that occurs just after lunch, from around 1 to 3 in the afternoon. The afternoon sleep period rarely lasts more than an hour and a half in adults. This desire for an afternoon siesta is encouraged in many cultures. And, just as there are preferred times for sleep, there is also a so-called "forbidden zone." For example, many people find it almost impossible to fall asleep between the hours of 7 and 9 p.m. As you'll see in Chapter 3, however, aspects of your Sleep Personality (what time you naturally prefer to go to bed and get up, to nap or not, and how long you sleep) play a role in the exact timing of your "preferred" and "forbidden" zones for sleep.

Accordingly, if no one told you how to plan your day, then you'd probably find that you're better able to concentrate on complex tasks in the morning, that you crave a nap in mid-afternoon, and that you feel pretty strong while exercising at about 5 p.m. Within an hour or two before midnight you'd be ready for a major sleep period. That's because your biological clock has set these rhythms in motion. You can work around them if you have to, or your own rhythms may be different enough to put you a few hours ahead or behind, as we'll discuss later. But all things being equal, most people would take a nap in mid-afternoon and go to bed before midnight if their schedules allowed it.

Timing Is Everything

The human biological clock—the SCN—is located right near the optic chiasm. The optic chiasm is the junction box where the pathways from the two eyes merge and cross over on their way to the brain, carrying visual information about the outside world, including information about light and dark. The SCN gathers information from a special bundle of nerves within the optic pathways and uses it to keep the body more or less synchronized—or entrained—to the environmental 24-hour cycle of light and dark. You can think of information about light and dark as a kind of force that nudges the biological clock and tries to keep it in step with the world around us.

In fact, it's important to note that the human body does not run on exactly a 24-hour day (hence the "about a day" definition discussed above), but usually on a slightly longer schedule. When it comes to the sleep/wake cycle, human participants in free-running experiments (in which they are protected from all outside stimuli including light and dark cycles) establish a day of between 24.2 to 25.5 hours, or almost an hour longer on average than the regular day. Every day they live under such conditions, their bedtimes shift later by an extra hour, so that by two weeks into the experiment, most participants are

about a half a day out of synchrony with the outside
world. Such experiments help confirm that what helps us
maintain our daily 24-hour rhythms is exposure to light.
Indeed, sunlight, or any light if it is bright enough, acts
as the main timegiver, or *Zeitgeber*, for most species.

Words to Sleep By

Zeitgeber is a German term that means "timegiver." In
chronobiology, Zeitgeber refers to the specific external
influences that synchronize our internal circadian system.

Even humans appear to have more than one way to receive information about light and dark. While the eyes
serve as the primary entryway, recent studies indicate
that information about light might also reach the brain
through sensors located on skin cells or perhaps in the
blood. In fact, a recent study by Scott Campbell at Cornell
University found that shining a bright light on the back of
the knees (a highly vascular area) can reset the biological
clock. By applying lights to the knees for three hours during the night, the researchers caused the participants' biological clocks to shift back or forward by a few hours. As
we'll show you in Chapter 6, any light of sufficient intensity can cause your body clock to move forward or back-
ward, depending on when you are exposed to it.

Setting Your Clock

Although light is our primary Zeitgeber, and our biological clock is a strong motivator for our physiological activities and behavior, we aren't forced to follow either one.
Instead, you're able to override your biological disposition

and willfully shift your bedtimes and wake-up times to accommodate changes in your daily schedule, at least on an occasional basis. It isn't always easy to do so, and some people feel the ill effects of such a shift almost immediately. Clearly, however, you aren't forced to go to sleep or wake up at a set time, at least not biologically speaking.

Fortunately, you get help in maintaining a fairly consistent schedule despite your personal, internal clock, not only from the light/dark Zeitgeber, but from a host of other timegivers as well. The timing of meals, the regularly scheduled exercise routine, the social schedules imposed by work, family, and friends—all of these familiar activities provide a sense of time that keeps the biological clock's pendulum swinging in the appropriate rhythm.

As synchronized as our biological and social Zeitgebers keep us as a society, however, a wide variety of individual differences in rhythms exists from one person to the next. Most are barely noticeable, but two groups of people— those who consistently crave the morning light and those who love to burn the midnight oil—illustrate just how much of a difference the biological clock can make on the way we feel every day.

Are You Catching the Worm or Burning Midnight Oil?

As you might have guessed, larks and owls have a different cycle in their circadian rhythms, with the owls peaking about two hours later than their lark counterparts. This difference occurs in many physical and mental rhythms, including the daily rise and fall of body temperature and the increase and decrease in hormone levels.

Set Your Alarm!

If you consistently wake up in the morning feeling tired and out-of-sorts without knowing why, you may need to see a sleep specialist to track down what really happens as you sleep. Even if you don't remember waking up, something internal or external could be disturbing your sleep without your being aware of it.

Psychologically, the difference in rhythms is even greater than this biological shift indicates. True larks adore the morning—breakfast tends to be their favorite meal of the day—they are alert and creative early in the day, and they usually spend quiet evenings before going to bed on the early side. Owls, on the other hand, often spurn breakfast (though they usually require caffeine to get them up and running) and only truly blossom as the day progresses. Needless to say, such strong preferences may lead to difficulties with job performance or other responsibilities. A lark who must work the night shift, for instance, is apt to be miserable—and perhaps poor at his or her job. And a night owl might be more than a little cranky if he or she has to drive the morning carpool. We'll discuss Larks and Owls—and help you discover which bird you are—in Chapter 3. For now, let's take a look at a related aspect of your internal clock: the natural sleep cycles.

The Rhythms of the Night

William Shakespeare once described sleep as "nature's soft nurse," and who among us would argue with him? Nothing feels better after a hard day of living than falling into the sweet oblivion of sleep, then waking up feeling refreshed, renewed, and ready to enjoy the new day.

Despite its restful and restorative qualities, however, sleep is not a static, quiet activity. In fact, a lot happens within the brain while you're getting your nightly shut-eye: Even at the deepest level of sleep, there is only a moderate decrease in brain activity compared to a waking state. If all goes well, you emerge from sleep feeling restored. If something goes wrong, however, you could wake up feeling groggy, cranky, and out of sorts.

What goes on in the brain at night that allows you to get the rest you need? You might just be surprised at how complex your sleep system really is.

The Stages of Sleep

Sleep has two basic components: a non-Rapid Eye Movement (abbreviated NREM) sleep and Rapid Eye Movement (REM) sleep, during which most dreaming occurs. NREM sleep is further divided into four stages of various intensities. These stages recur four or five times in an orderly progression during the average eight hours of sleep. Please note, however, that the length of time spent in each stage of sleep, and total sleep time, changes at different stages of life, a fact we'll discuss in more depth in Part 4.

The time from sleep onset to the end of the first REM sleep is called the first "sleep cycle," and the time from then to the end of the next REM sleep is the second sleep cycle. There are usually about four or five sleep cycles a night—each lasting about 90 to 100 minutes per cycle. The amount of each sleep stage within a cycle changes throughout the night. In the first half of the night there is more deep sleep (NREM Stages 3 and 4); and in the second half, REM takes over, making up more and more of each sleep cycle. Your final REM episode can last up to 30 minutes or more.

The Dream of REM

REM sleep is also known as "paradoxical" sleep, and for good reason. First, the brain is working so hard that it's

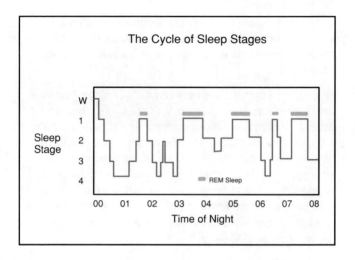

You cycle through the four sleep stages and a period of REM sleep several times each night, with each cycle taking about 90 to 100 minutes.

almost like being awake. Second, the brain is very active but the body is motionless. As mentioned in Chapter 1, a nerve center in the brain keeps muscles in a state of near paralysis during REM sleep. If this did not occur, you'd be acting out your dreams while still unconscious.

For centuries, artists and philosophers have pondered the meaning of dreams; and more recently, scientists and physicians have searched for the medical purpose and consequences of dreams. An important step along the way took place in 1953, when scientist Nathaniel Kleitman observed his sleeping son and saw that the child's eyes periodically moved about, back and forth, as if he were watching a silent movie inside his head. Digging out an old EEG machine from the basement of the University of Chicago where he studied, Kleitman recorded his son's brain waves while he slept. The readings revealed a brain so active it might as well have been awake. He and his colleagues named this sleep "Rapid Eye Movement" sleep, or REM sleep.

Suspecting a connection between REM sleep and dreaming, Kleitmann, sleep pioneer William C. Dement, and other researchers set about proving that theory the only way possible: In study after study, they woke people out of REM sleep and asked them about their dreams. The answers confirmed it: Between 80 and 95 percent of REM sleepers reported vivid dreams, compared to only 7 percent of those woken from NREM sleep. (Yes, you do occasionally dream while in other sleep stages, but the primary dream stage is REM sleep.)

During REM sleep, then, we're awake within ourselves, thinking and performing in an altered state. As you may know, some philosophers, psychiatrists, and artists believe dreams represent our minds and souls. In addition to the metaphysical meaning of dreams, however, REM sleep apparently serves a biological purpose. What that purpose is and why it developed on the other hand, remain questions in need of answers.

Rest Easy

Time your naps. If you need to get rid of your drowsiness, for best results take a 15- or 20-minute nap—just long enough to reach Stage 2 sleep, but not long enough to reach the deepest sleep. A nap of this length will suffice if you're pressed for time, but if you can afford it, nap for about 90 minutes, which will take you through one whole sleep cycle. That way, you might even get in an interesting dream!

One theory is that REM sleep helps consolidate memory and emotion. We know, for instance, that blood flow during REM sleep rises sharply in several brain areas linked to the processing of memories and emotional experiences. Blood flow declines, on the other hand, in areas involved in complex reasoning and language, located at the front of the brain.

Sleep studies performed at the Weizmann Institute in Israel seem to confirm this theory. Subjects were shown various objects on a computer screen and then tested later for recall. After depriving some of the subjects of REM sleep, researchers found that memory recall was impaired in that group, while the subjects who slept uninterrupted had no changes in performance.

Other studies supporting the memory consolidation connection suggest the involvement of a brain chemical called acetylcholine in the process. Known for its role in the process of memory (it is produced by the same brain cells damaged in memory disorders like Alzheimer's disease) and found throughout the body, acetylcholine levels surge during REM sleep, but not in other sleep stages.

In any case, the need for REM sleep is certain: If deprived of it for one or more nights, you'll wake up feeling irritable and unable to concentrate. Then you'll "reimburse" yourself by dreaming more the next time you get a full night's sleep. In fact, on the following nights, your dreaming will start sooner and last much longer, consuming a greater percentage of total sleep time than usual.

The same can be said for the other stages of sleep, collectively known as NREM. As much as we need to dream, we also need to heal and to restore. If deprived of Stages 3 and 4 sleep, you'll wake up feeling extremely sleepy the next day, no matter how much light sleep and REM sleep you've enjoyed.

The Depth of Non-REM

Your body is relaxed, your brain is at rest, and you're able to move around a bit to get more comfortable without waking up: Now this is what sleep is *really* supposed to be like, isn't it? NREM sleep, which accounts for about 80 percent of the total sleep time of the average young adult, appears to restore the body in the same way that REM sleep may help restore the brain and the emotions.

First, and perhaps most important, the body truly rests during NREM sleep. All physiological functions—body temperature, blood pressure, heart rate, respiration rate, digestion, urinary function, and brain activity—slow down. Although you're able to move about (the average person shifts body position more than 30 times a night), muscles are relaxed. Interestingly enough, studies indicate that our muscles might receive just as much relaxation and repair during simple rest periods, and that the state of unconsciousness we call sleep may not be necessary for this purpose. It seems that our brains need sleep far more than our bodies do—no matter how good it feels to hit the sheets after a hard day of physical work and play!

In addition, your body produces a much-needed hormone during sleep—one that helps repair and maintain your muscles and bones. During Stages 3 and 4 of NREM sleep, the body receives almost all its daily dose of an important hormone called human growth hormone (HGH). HGH is secreted by the pituitary, an endocrine gland located at the base of the brain. A protein hormone, HGH promotes the growth, maintenance, and repair of muscles and bones by facilitating the use of amino acids, the essential building blocks of protein. Although the actual synthesis of protein and repair of muscles may take place both during the day and at night, the body does require NREM sleep in order to release the hormone in the first place.

In the end, then, it's clear that both main phases of sleep—REM and NREM—are necessary for the maintenance of good health and good cheer.

Your Need for Sleep

Allan Hobson, one of the leading neurobiologists studying sleep today, wrote, "Nature is much too economical to waste hours of biological time doing nothing but simply saving energy and idling the brain. . . A night of sleep is as much preparation for the subsequent day's activity as recovery from that of the previous day."

Without question, sleep is as important to your health as proper nutrition and regular exercise—and quality of sleep appears to be just as important as quantity. Indeed, even if you sleep for eight or nine hours, you may still suffer from the effects of too little sleep if you spend too much time in the lighter stages of sleep and not enough in the deeper stages and REM periods. Or perhaps you suffer from one of the many sleep disorders, such as sleep apnea or Periodic Leg Movements (discussed in Chapter 10), that can disrupt you—and your partner, perhaps—without your being aware of the problem. In some cases, you might be able to track down the culprit yourself, using the tips we give you in the coming chapters. In other cases, you may need the help of a qualified professional trained in the fine art of sleep medicine.

Chapter 3

What Kind of Sleeper Are You?

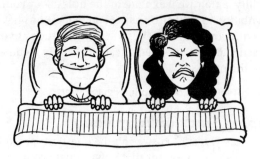

In This Chapter

➤ Determine your sleep patterns
➤ Identify your "Circadian Type"
➤ Explore your "Nap-Ability"
➤ Make your "Sleep Personality" work for you

Do you realize that you have a "Sleep Personality" all your own? Your Sleep Personality consists of certain natural tendencies that determine to a large degree when and how well you sleep. In a series of quizzes in this chapter, you'll find out all about yours. First, you'll find out your "Circadian Type"—that is, if you're naturally a morning or a night person. You'll also discover your "Flex-Ability," or how well you can adapt to changes that disrupt your natural rhythms. The next quiz will identify your "Sleep Type"—whether you're a long or short sleeper—by focusing on how much total sleep you need both during your major sleep period (usually occurring at night) and throughout the day (in the form of naps). This aspect of your Sleep Personality relates as well to your napping capability, a trait we'll explore in the quiz about your "Nap-Ability." You'll also answer some questions having to do with your nighttime responsibilities, such as your work schedule or your need to care for family members during the night.

We've got a lot to cover, so let's get started.

Keeping Track of Your Sleep

Even before you start answering the questions posed in the quizzes, it's important that you evaluate your current sleep patterns. Frankly, sleep is an activity most of us take for granted, even when we know we could probably get more, or better quality, sleep. To help you more fully understand your own sleep patterns, we've designed a Sleep Log for you to fill in for a week or two—or longer if you work an irregular schedule.

In this log, you'll record several aspects of your sleep life: the time you get into bed, when you turn off the lights, the estimated length of time you lay in bed before you actually fall asleep, the estimated number and duration of any awakenings, the time you wake up, the time you get out of bed, and the frequency and duration of naps. To keep a Sleep Log for a week or two, you'll need copies of the log, a pen or pencil to keep by your bed, and an accurate, readable bedside clock.

Set Your Alarm!

Be careful not to become addicted to clock-watching during the night. The more concerned you are about what time it is—and how little you've slept—the more anxious you'll become, making it even more difficult for you to fall asleep.

Just before you turn out the lights, mark down the time. However—and this is important—you should avoid looking at the clock during the night after you check to see what time it is at Lights Out. If you have trouble sleeping—and we'll assume you do since you're reading this book—you shouldn't look at the clock until you're fully awake and ready to roll out of bed in the morning.

Then, when you wake up in the morning, fill out the rest of the log. Try to be as accurate as you can about how long it took you to actually fall asleep after Lights Out, and be sure to make careful note of if and when you woke up during the night and how long it took you to get back to sleep. Another important criterion for you to consider is your sleep quality. How do you think you slept? Did you stay awake for a long period of time, anxious and distressed? Did you toss and turn? Wake up constantly? Were you exhausted in the morning? You may find it helpful to rate your sleep quality on a scale of one to six, with one being terrible and six being excellent.

You'll also want to track how many hours each day you work—outside or inside the home—and how many hours are spent simply relaxing, as well as how often and for how long you nap during the day. This will help you calculate how much total sleep you need in any 24-hour period, and when your need for a nap occurs most often.

Your Sleep Log

Date _____

Worktime _____

Playtime _____

Bedtime _____

Lights Out _____

Sleep Onset _____

Awakenings:

Number/Length _____

Wake-Up Time _____

Rise Time _____

Sleep Quality (1 = terrible, 2 = poor, 3 = fair, 4 = good, 5 = very good, 6 = excellent) _____

Nap Time/Duration _____

Once you've kept your Sleep Log for a few weeks, you can start to figure out what your natural sleep/wake rhythm is and how much sleep you really need. This rhythm will become even clearer as you take the following quizzes.

Your Circadian and Flex-Ability Profile

The "morning person" (the Lark) is the kind of person who's up with the sun, bustling about, and getting her best work done before lunch. The "night person" (the Owl) is somebody who flourishes in the afternoon and evening and wouldn't care if he never saw the early morning dew again. The intermediate person—whom we call the "Regular Robin"—doesn't go to either extreme, but can cope with early mornings and late nights as the need arises.

You know who you are. Or do you? Have you ever really thought about what part of the day truly suits you or when your body would prefer to sleep? We'll help you answer those questions here.

Are You a Lark or an Owl?

This quiz will help sort out the Larks and Owls from the Regular Robins. Consider each question with care and, if need be, check back through your Sleep Log.

Your Circadian Identity

Choose the answer that best relates to your own sleep experience.

1. What time would you get up if you were entirely free to plan your day?

   1 point: Before 7 a.m.

   2 points: 7–9 a.m.

   3 points: After 9 a.m.

2. How easy is it for you to get up on workdays?

   1 point: Fairly easy

   2 points: Moderately difficult/depends on the day

   3 points: Very difficult

3. How alert do you feel during the first 30 minutes after you get up in the morning?

   1 point: Alert/fresh

   2 points: Varies

   3 points: Sleepy/tired

4. What time would you go to bed if it were completely up to you?

   1 point: Before 10:30 p.m.

   2 points: 10:30 p.m.–midnight

   3 points: After midnight

5. How sleepy/tired are you 1½ hours before going to bed during the workweek?

   1 point: Very tired/ready to fall asleep

   2 points: Moderately tired/depends on the day

   3 points: Not very tired

6. When you've stayed up later than usual (had a late evening), when do you wake up the next morning (assuming you didn't have any alcohol)?

   1 point: At your usual time, with a desire to get out of bed

   2 points: Varies

   3 points: Later than usual, with a desire to fall back asleep

To score this quiz, simply add up your points. You'll come up with a score between 6 and 18. Plot this score on the Circadian Type/Flex-Ability Profile on the following page. Generally speaking, the lower your number, the more of a morning person you are.

How Flexible are You?

Are you one of those people who needs to be in bed at the same time every night and has to get your regular amount of sleep or you're just not yourself the next day? Or can you adapt fairly easily to changes in your sleep schedule? Take this quiz to find out.

Your Flex-Ability Quotient

1. When you're feeling drowsy, can you easily overcome it if there is something important you have to do?

1 point: Rarely

2 points: Sometimes

3 points: Usually

2. When you have to do something important in the middle of the night, can you do it almost as easily as you could at a more normal time of the day?

   1 point: Rarely

   2 points: Sometimes

   3 points: Usually

3. Do you enjoy working at unusual times of the day or night?

   1 point: Rarely

   2 points: Sometimes

   3 points: Usually

4. If you have a lot to do, can you stay up late or get up very early to finish it without feeling too tired?

   1 point: Rarely

   2 points: Sometimes

   3 points: Usually

5. Do you find it as easy to work late at night as you do earlier in the day?

   1 point: Rarely

   2 points: Sometimes

   3 points: Usually

6. Do you find it fairly easy to sleep whenever you want to?

   1 point: Rarely

   2 points: Sometimes

   3 points: Usually

Again, total your score using the point tallies indicated. Generally speaking, the lower your score, the more rigid or inflexible you are about your sleep needs. The higher your score, the more able you are to adapt to outside demands on your time and energy.

Taken together, your scores on these two quizzes place you within a section of the Circadian/Flex-Ability Type Profile that is shown in the following figure. As we've laid it out here, most people fall into one of three general categories: Rigid Lark, Regular Robin, or Flexible Owl.

Where did your score put you? If you're someone who rises promptly at 6 a.m. every morning—even when on vacation—and if you have a lot of trouble functioning after your normal bedtime, you're probably in the *"Rigid Lark"* category.

Words to Sleep By

A **Rigid Lark** is someone whose natural sleep pattern gets her up very early in the morning and makes it very difficult for her to sleep in, even if she is forced to stay up past her normal bedtime.

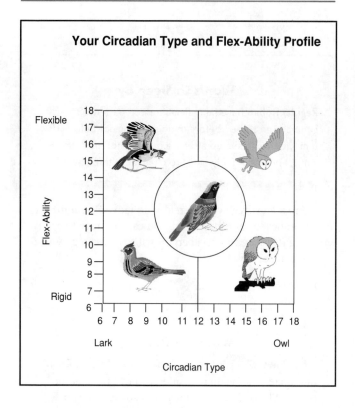

Your Circadian Type and Flex-Ability Profile

Plot your scores from the Circadian and Flex-Ability quizzes on this chart. The closer you are to the middle of the chart, the more of a Regular Robin you tend to be. The closer to the top of the chart, the more flexible you are, and the farther left your score puts you, the more Lark tendencies you have.

You're a *Regular Robin* if you usually to go to bed between 10 p.m. and midnight, generally wake up between 6 and 8 a.m., and can manage to function fairly well on either end of the spectrum if circumstances warrant it.

Words to Sleep By

Regular Robins have fairly flexible sleep patterns. They generally go to bed before midnight (but not before 10 p.m.), usually wake up after 6 a.m. (but not after, say, 8 a.m.), and adapt fairly easily to changes in this schedule.

If you're a *Flexible Owl*, you really do crave the night and function best after dinner, but you can manage to adjust your regular schedule to keep up with the average 9-to-5 world if necessary.

Words to Sleep By

A **Flexible Owl** is your good old-fashioned "night person" who prefers staying up until after midnight (and maybe even until 1 or 2 a.m.), but who can adapt to a 9-to-5 routine if need be.

Here are a few other examples of type-specific behavior and preferences based on these profiles:

If you're a Rigid Lark, you

➤ Would have a hard time staying up late at night even if you were invited to a Beatles midnight reunion, never mind having to work on your company's annual report

➤ Are a very poor candidate for night-shift work

➤ Might need to learn some special napping strategies if you become sleep-deprived

If you're a Regular Robin, you

➤ May have a preference for working in the morning or evening, but you're not *adamant* about it (like some people!)

➤ Are likely to be rather intolerant of the sleep habits and problems of your Rigid Lark or Flexible Owl counterparts

➤ Can usually follow general prescriptions for getting a good night's sleep

If you're a Flexible Owl, you

➤ Prefer the night, and resist working and playing too early in the morning

➤ Are an ideal candidate for night-shift work

➤ May get into trouble if you have morning responsibilities but allow yourself to stay up too late at night

As you can see, your natural rhythms have a great deal of influence not only on the way you sleep, but also on how well your body and mind function throughout the day. In the chapters to come, we'll explore how you can use what you know about your Circadian/Flex-Ability Profile to help solve your sleep problems and to help you function better throughout your day and night.

Your Sleep Type and Nap-Ability Profile

The next two quizzes determine how much you want (and probably need) to sleep and how well and how often you nap. Once you determine the answer to those questions, you'll have a greater understanding of what your optimal sleep/wake pattern should be throughout your day.

How Long Are You "Out?"

Some people just love to sleep: eight, nine, even ten hours of shut-eye a night is perfect for their particular physiological make-up. Other people jump out of bed after what their longer-sleeping counterparts might consider a catnap, but they feel refreshed and rested enough to meet the challenges of the day. To find out which category you fit into, take the following quiz.

Your Sleep Type

Answer each question with one of the following:

a.	less than 5 hours	1 point
b.	5–6 hours	2 points
c.	6–7 hours	3 points
d.	7–8 hours	4 points
e.	8–9 hours	5 points
f.	9–10 hours	6 points
g.	10–11 hours	7 points
h.	more than 11 hours	8 points

1. How many total hours (night sleep plus daytime naps) of sleep do you usually get per working day? _____

2. How many total hours of sleep do you usually get per day (night sleep plus daytime naps) on your days off? _____

3. How many hours of total sleep do you get when you're on vacation? _____

4. How many hours would you sleep when you're not sleep-deprived (when you've had one or more nights of optimal sleep) and can go to bed and wake up when you want to? _____

5. How many hours of sleep do you think you need in order to function at your best the next day? _____

Add up your score using the values assigned to each letter at the beginning of the quiz. Your score will fall between 5 and 40 points, with a score of 5 identifying you as an extremely short sleeper and a score of 40 as an extremely long sleeper.

Are You a Napper?

Are you one of those people who can close his eyes for 10 minutes, drift off to dreamland, and then wake up refreshed? Have you made a one- to two-hour siesta a regular part of your day? Or is sleeping during the day difficult—if not impossible—for you? Take this quiz to find out how you score as a napper.

Test Your Nap-Ability

Check your Sleep Log if you need help answering the following questions.

1. Can you easily nap during the daytime when you are not particularly sleep-deprived?

   1 point: Rarely

   2 points: Sometimes

   3 points: Usually

2. Can you easily nap during the daytime to "catch up" on lost sleep, such as after one or more late nights?

   1 point: Rarely

   2 points: Sometimes

   3 points: Usually

3. On days off, do you take a daytime nap?

   1 point: Rarely

   2 points: Sometimes

   3 points: Usually

4. Do you feel refreshed after a daytime nap?

   1 point: Rarely

   2 points: Sometimes

   3 points: Usually

5. Do you use brief naps (less than 30 minutes) to sustain your alertness during an extended monotonous task (for example, driving a long distance) or when staying up all night?

   1 point: Rarely

   2 points: Sometimes

   3 points: Usually

Your total score for this quiz will fall between 5 and 15. The lower your score, the less able you are to nap. The higher your score, the more likely it is that napping forms an integral part of your daily sleep/wake pattern.

Once you find your scores on both these quizzes, plot the corresponding number on Your Sleep Type and Nap-Ability Profile, shown in the following figure.

Where did your score put you in this profile? Generally speaking, you're in the best shape if you fall into one of these three categories:

> ➤ **A long sleeper who does not nap.** This means that most of the time you get all the sleep you require

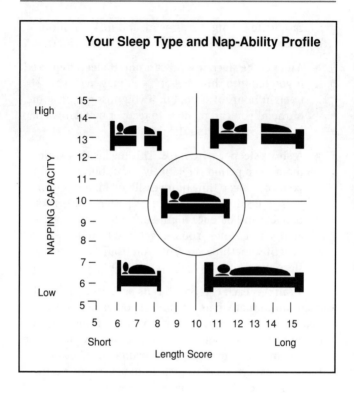

Your Sleep Type and Nap-Ability Profile

Plot your scores from the Sleep Type and Nap-Ability quizzes on this chart. The closer to the middle of the chart you fall, the more "average" your sleep patterns tend to be. If your score places you in the top half you like to nap and are able to do so easily—whether you're a short sleeper (on the left side of the chart) or a long sleeper (on the right side of the chart).

during your main sleep period (usually at night). Because you don't nap, you easily become sleep-deprived if something cuts short your main sleep period. This characteristic makes you a less-than-ideal candidate for night-shift work and makes it more likely that you'll suffer from jet lag when you travel.

➤ **An average sleeper who can nap if sleep-deprived.** If you fall into this category, you may need your six to eight hours of sleep, but if you miss out on some of them, you can manage to recover by taking a nap at some point during the day.

➤ **A short sleeper who naps.** This means that your main sleep period is relatively short, but you add to your total sleep time quite easily by taking one or more naps during the day. This pattern makes you a perfect candidate for night-shift work and travel across time zones. You can get into trouble, however, if something prevents you from catching up on sleep during the day.

As you can see, each category has its benefits and its risks. Keep in mind that whatever pattern you've developed probably works for you, as long as you feel rested and alert during your awake hours, feel that you sleep well, and are able to maintain your work/rest schedule. Just because some sleep experts seem to preach that everyone needs eight hours doesn't mean that you do.

The only exceptions to this general rule concern those of you who fall outside these three main categories. If you're a very short sleeper—someone who regularly gets less than five hours of sleep—who can't nap, for instance, you may well be sleep-deprived because of a clinical sleep disorder or medical problem. The same can be said if you're a very long sleeper—someone who regularly needs more than nine or ten hours of sleep—but who still needs to nap during the day on a regular basis. Some underlying medical problem or sleep disorder may be triggering this extreme need for sleep.

No matter how well adjusted you are to your sleep patterns and circadian rhythms, you're apt to be thrown off if you're required to do something important when your body expects to be asleep. The following quiz will help determine if you fall into that category.

Night Work 101

Would you just love to crawl into bed at 11 p.m. and sleep clear through 'til the alarm rings at 6:30—but you can't because other responsibilities keep you up all night or drag you from sleep on a regular basis? If so, you're not alone. Although we tend to think of "night work" as involving factories or all-night diners, many of you may be working through the night for other reasons altogether. Take this quiz to find out.

Your Night Work Evaluation

1. Do you work a fixed night shift?

   Yes ____ No ____

2. Does your work schedule require you to rotate from days to nights on a regular basis?

   Yes ____ No ____

3. Do you routinely work more than 60 hours per week?

   Yes ____ No ____

4. Do you have a family member, such as an infant or ailing parent, who requires your attention during the overnight hours on a regular basis?

   Yes ____ No ____

5. Do you have a second job in addition to your full-time occupation?

   Yes ____ No ____

If you answered yes to one or more of these questions, you should probably go right ahead and read Chapter 12 for information about sleep solutions for your situation.

That said, it bears repeating that if you wake up feeling rested after spending a peaceful night asleep, your life and your sleep needs are balanced—you're able to sleep when your body craves it, and you wake up having slept enough to function well throughout your day.

So Who Are You, Anyway?

What did you learn about your Sleep Personality in this chapter? Did you find out that the way your life is structured coincides with your natural sleep rhythms, or is there a problem in that area? If you've found that you have extreme Lark or Owl tendencies, you may want to skip ahead and read Chapter 10 for some suggestions tailored just for you. Do you need some tips on napping because your nighttime responsibilities interfere with your ability to get enough sleep? Then read Chapter 8.

As you know, many books about sleep fail to consider individual needs and preferences when it comes to discussing solutions to sleep problems and other advice. You'll see that throughout this text, we offer you specific advice targeted to meet the needs of your particular Sleep Personality. In the meantime, it's time to see what might be interfering with your ability to get the sleep you need— no matter what your Sleep Personality might be. Chapter 4 will help pin down what's keeping you up at night.

What's Keeping You Up at Night?

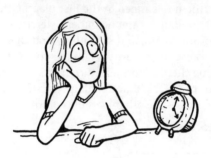

In This Chapter

➤ Understanding insomnia

➤ Tracking down a medical problem or sleep disorder

➤ Identifying lifestyle culprits

Insomnia—the endless stretch of hours awake in the dark, exhausted, anxious, frustrated. Days spent fighting fatigue in numbing exhaustion. If you're reading this book because you're suffering with insomnia, you know just how physically and emotionally debilitating it can be.

The good news is that insomnia is often a treatable condition, one that can be alleviated—if not solved—by getting the medical help you need and/or by making changes in the way you live during the day and in the environment you create for sleep. We'll discuss those changes in the chapters to come. In the meantime, let's explore the world of insomnia and what it really looks like.

What Kind of Insomniac Are You?

Insomnia isn't one simple condition with just one set
of causes, symptoms, and solutions. Some people have
trouble sleeping because they take medication that triggers the "wake centers" in the brain or because the discomfort of a chronic illness wakes them in the night, or
doesn't let them fall asleep in the first place. Other insomniacs drink too much caffeine, others exercise too close to
bedtime (or not at all), and still others find themselves up
at night because their mattress fails to support their lower
back, leaving them to toss and turn in discomfort
throughout the night. Emotional upsets, stress overload,
and mild illnesses are other possible culprits.

Rest Easy

Be open to a trial-and-error approach to solving your
sleep problem. Solving it may require you to evaluate
many aspects of your sleeping and waking life, and then
making one or more changes until you find yourself
sleeping better. For more help, visit our Web site at
www.goodsleep.com.

Some people have trouble with falling asleep, others with
staying asleep, and still others with waking up too early.
Many people wake up tired because they don't time their
sleep properly, thereby interrupting a sleep cycle. And
then there are the people who have an occasional bad
night of sleep, others who have spells of a few weeks or
months when sleep is difficult, and still others whose
sleep problems become chronic.

We'll help you sort out some of the reasons you might
be having a tough time getting enough sleep later in

this chapter. In the meantime, you may be surprised to learn how very different you may be from your insomniac counterparts, for insomnia does indeed come in all shapes and sizes.

Fortunately, there are very few people—even those who define themselves as helpless insomniacs—who *never* go to sleep throughout an entire night. Generally speaking, insomniacs fall into one of three categories:

➤ **Delayed sleepers** have trouble falling asleep once they get into bed. Generally speaking, Owls tend to develop this problem more often than Larks, especially when they're trying to get to sleep earlier than usual in order to wake up earlier.

➤ **Frequent awakeners** are disturbed from sleep often several times during the night. In most cases, stress and anxiety are the causes, but a sleep disorder like apnea or a medical problem like chronic pain may also trigger this type of insomnia.

➤ **Early awakeners** find themselves waking up very early in the morning—generally before 5 a.m.— before having had enough sleep. Larks tend to find themselves in this situation more often than their Owl counterparts, especially as they start to become tired and fall asleep earlier in the evening to make up for the loss of sleep in the morning. By getting up and switching on the lights, they compound the problem by reprogramming their bodies to wake up earlier and earlier on successive mornings. It's important to note as well that early awakening is one of the hallmark signs of depression, a possibility you and your doctor should consider if you find yourself often waking up too early.

Unfortunately, once the natural patterns of "Owls" and "Larks" become disrupted, chronic sleep deprivation can result, especially if these natural patterns are very rigid.

Sleep Personality Pitfalls

Take Oliver, for instance. Oliver is naturally an extreme Owl. In the best of all possible worlds, Oliver would stay awake until 2 a.m. and sleep until 8 or 9 in the morning (he feels best on about six hours of sleep per night). Oliver prefers to work at tasks that take the most concentration between 10 p.m. and 1 a.m. However, he does find it relatively easy to shift his bedtime back about two hours, so that he falls asleep about midnight and wakes up at 6 or 7 a.m. This would give him plenty of time to get to work by 10 a.m. or so. Since Oliver works for a company that allows its employees to make their own hours most of the time, Oliver's sleep pattern works well for him.

Oliver can easily get into trouble, however, if he is called into an early morning meeting—one that convenes at 8 or 9 a.m. If he is unable to fall asleep earlier than usual the night before, he will wake up feeling tired in the morning and drag through the day. By 8 or 9 p.m. he'll be so exhausted that he will fall asleep at that time. If he could sleep straight through to morning, it would be okay, but instead, he usually wakes up—fresh as a daisy—at midnight and then can't fall asleep again until near dawn. He'll also get into the same kind of trouble if he loses sight of the time and simply works until his natural sleep rhythm kicks in, which could be as late as 2 or 3 a.m.

Once such a pattern is established, the only way Oliver can break it is by making sure that he naps for just an hour around 8 p.m. and then works until his regular sleep time of midnight or so. If he then sleeps through to his regular wake-up time of 6 or 7 a.m., he'll be back on his regular schedule.

Letitia, on the other hand, is a Lark, and a rather rigid one to boot. Lights out for Letitia is usually around 10 p.m. and her wake-up time around 4 a.m. (four complete

90-minute sleep cycles). Having very good Nap-Ability, Letitia easily adds to her sleep during the day by taking either a few 10-minute catnaps or, if she's feeling especially sleep-deprived, a full hour-and-a-half nap (one full sleep cycle).

Letitia can get into trouble with her sleep patterns, however, if something keeps her up much later than normal. Being a Rigid Lark, Letitia won't naturally continue to sleep until she gets her regular six hours, but instead will wake up promptly at 4 a.m. no matter how little she's slept. If she can't catch a nap during the workday, she'll end up being too tired and edgy to go to sleep earlier than her usual time. The fact that she usually grabs more sugar snacks and caffeinated beverages during the day to give her a little boost doesn't help either.

Once she becomes overtired and stressed, Letitia finds herself waking up earlier and earlier—sometimes as early as 3 a.m.—and cutting back more and more on her sleep until she's exhausted. Only by taking a long, restful one-and-a-half-hour nap at least five hours before her normal bedtime (so as not to prevent her from falling asleep) can she break out of this cycle that would eventually lead to chronic insomnia. Interestingly, once she has taken such a nap, she finds she has reset her sleep/wake cycle and that night will stay up an extra half-hour but sleep through to 5:30 or 6 a.m. (that is, she'll get five instead of four full sleep cycles). Eventually, Letitia will go back to her normal 10 p.m. to 4 a.m. schedule.

Do you recognize yourself in either Oliver (the Owl) or Letitia (the Lark)? Could your sleep problem be linked to a disruption in your natural rhythm? Of course, the examples cited here are just two of the many types of insomnia patterns—and we'll be describing others as we go along. If you're a Regular Robin, for instance, a disruption on either end of your day can lead to difficulties.

In any case, it's important for you to evaluate your sleep patterns in this way as you consider the source of your current difficulties—and we'll remind you of that approach often. In most cases of mild to moderate sleep difficulties, lifestyle issues—including time-zone travel, shift work, diet and exercise habits, and stress levels—are the likely culprits. We'll discuss those problems and their solutions in other chapters.

For now, though, we want to stress that if you have a stubborn sleep problem and haven't had a recent checkup with your primary physician, now is the time to make that appointment.

The Medical Route

Chronic pain, heart disease, stomach ulcers, and many other medical illnesses can disrupt your sleep by increasing the amount of time it takes to fall asleep, by increasing the number of times you wake up during the night, and by decreasing your overall depth of sleep throughout the night. The good news is that once the underlying problem is identified and treated, the sleep problem often dissipates as well. The bad news is that certain medications designed to treat these very same conditions could end up upsetting your sleep. That's why it's essential that you talk with your doctor about your sleep patterns, along with any other medical symptoms you experience, on a regular basis.

Clearly, it goes far beyond the scope of this book to explore the full range of sleep-related medical issues. What we'll do, however, is give you a list of the most common medical conditions affecting sleep so that you can discuss them with your doctor. They include:

➤ **Arthritis.** Arthritis is a general term for more than 100 different conditions that cause inflammation—and usually swelling and pain—of the joints. In all forms of arthritis, the pain often becomes worse at night, which increases the time spent awake in bed and the amount of light sleep during the night. Unfortunately, a vicious circle often ensues, since the stress of insomnia often worsens the pain of some forms of arthritis.

➤ **Headaches.** Headaches come in many forms and have many different causes. There are the throbbing migraines, the aching sinus headaches, the run-of-the-mill tension headaches, and a host of others. Most of the time, headaches are not life threatening and will pass on their own or with the aid of analgesics or other medication. If you have severe headaches that disturb your sleep, however, it's important to see your doctor for an evaluation.

➤ **Frequent urination.** Any condition that sends you to the bathroom several times a night—a condition called *nocturia*—will disrupt your sleep, including urinary tract infections, urinary incontinence and, in men, an enlarged prostate gland.

Set Your Alarm!

Don't assume that a need to urinate is what actually wakes you up during the night. A 1997 study in the *Journal of the American Medical Association* showed that other sleep problems, particularly sleep apnea, caused the initial awakening in a group of older adults, who only then felt the need to urinate. Talk to your doctor if you have this problem.

➤ **Breathing problems.** It stands to reason that any medical condition that interferes with breathing would disrupt sleep. Such conditions include asthma, emphysema and other chronic lung conditions, and allergies. They often result in increased wakefulness and more time spent in lighter sleep.

➤ **Heart disease.** Any form of heart disease, including angina (severe chest pain that occurs when the oxygen supply to the heart is interrupted), coronary artery disease, and congestive heart disease can cause sleep problems. In addition, the medication used to treat these conditions can also disturb sleep. Some may also trigger chronic nightmares.

➤ **Stomach problems.** Difficulty getting to sleep, fragmented sleep, frequent awakenings. . .you name the sleep problem, and a gastrointestinal tract problem, such as peptic ulcer disease and gastroesophogeal reflux—commonly known as heartburn—may be the cause of it.

➤ **Allergies.** Who could sleep with an itchy rash, a raspy cough, or a headache caused by stuffed sinuses? All these allergy-related symptoms, and others, can disrupt sleep patterns—and so can the drugs used to treat them.

➤ **Nervous system disorders.** Any condition that involves a disruption of brain chemistry can also disrupt sleep, including Parkinson's disease, epilepsy, muscular dystrophy, Tourette's syndrome, Huntington's chorea, dystonia and others. These conditions increase the number of awakenings, shifts between the stages of sleep, and the amount of time spent in light rather than deep sleep. And as is true for so many other medical conditions, the medications used to treat nervous system disorders may also disturb sleep.

➤ **Menstruation, pregnancy, and menopause.**
Thanks to the hormone fluctuations they experience, women have special problems with sleep. Changing hormone levels during the week before menstruation, for instance, can increase the time it takes to go to sleep or can cause multiple awakenings.

➤ **Depression.** Along with overwhelming feelings of despair, worthlessness, and guilt, depression also causes physical symptoms that can include weight loss or weight gain, gastrointestinal problems, and changes in sleep patterns. Usually people with depression suffer from very early morning awakenings, but sometimes people with depression also have trouble getting to sleep. People with Seasonal Affective Disorder (SAD), a type of depression that usually occurs in the fall and winter months when day lengths are shorter, tend to sleep too much because they lack exposure to sufficient bright light.

Rest Easy

If you have trouble sleeping after suffering an emotional trauma, talk to your doctor. Under this type of special circumstance, taking medication under close medical supervision may be appropriate. Otherwise, your ability to cope with the trauma may well become hampered by the effects of sleep deprivation.

➤ **Anxiety disorders.** People with anxiety have trouble falling and then staying asleep, and they experience fragmented and unrefreshing sleep.

➤ **Medications to treat medical conditions.** A whole host of drugs used to treat a very wide range of medical and psychiatric conditions can make it difficult for you to sleep well. At the same time, there are medications that actually promote sleep, or at least make you sleepy, but too often, these effects occur at the wrong time (like while you're driving or trying to concentrate). It's essential that you talk to your doctor about every medicine you take and how it may be affecting your ability to get a good night's sleep. If there's a connection between that drug and your sleep problem, there's a good chance your doctor can find an equally effective drug that will not cause this debilitating side effect.

Disordered Sleep: The Clinical Story

In addition to the medical conditions and types of medication that indirectly cause sleep problems, there are several disorders directly related to sleep—and millions of Americans suffer from one or more of them without being aware of it. In fact, the National Commission on Sleep Disorders Research estimates that 95 percent of people with sleep disorders are undiagnosed and untreated.

If you're one of them, your problem may warrant a visit to a sleep lab. There, sleep specialists will run a series of tests to determine the underlying cause. In the pages to come, we discuss some of the conditions they'll check you for.

Loud and Not So Clear

Snoring and Obstructive Sleep Apnea are two different, but often related, conditions that can interfere with proper sleep. Take the following quiz to see if you might be affected by one or both of them.

1. I know or have been told that I snore loudly.
   True _____ False _____

2. I chronically feel tired.
   True _____ False _____

3. My partner has heard me gasping for breath, or has heard me stop breathing for more than a few seconds while I sleep.
   True _____ False _____

If you answered "true" to the first question, you already know who you are—a snorer! If you've been having trouble sleeping, or don't feel rested during the day, your snoring may be waking you up or keeping you from sleeping deeply. Your partner (if you have one) may also be suffering because your snoring keeps him or her up at night.

A "true" response to questions 2 and 3, especially if you also answered "true" to the first question, strongly indicates that you suffer from a related disorder called Obstructive Sleep Apnea. In sleep apnea, your airways collapse, which causes periodic reductions or complete interruptions in airflow during sleep. In other words, you stop breathing while you are asleep until the brain finally gets the message that the body needs more oxygen. At that point, you wake up, usually snorting and gasping for air, and most of the time not realizing that you're doing so. You drift back to sleep quickly, and the problem starts all over again—in fact, it can happen hundreds of times a night. We'll discuss this condition in Chapter 9.

Up in the Night

Millions of Americans don't assume the common posture for sleep—eyes closed with the body relatively still and supine. Instead, they move about freely—far too freely—during the night, preventing themselves and often their partners from getting a good night's sleep. See if you're one of them by answering the following questions.

1. I often experience a "creepy crawly" feeling or other unusual sensation in my lower legs in the evening before I go to sleep.
   True _____ False _____

2. I often have to get out of bed or shake my leg to relieve pain or discomfort.
   True _____ False _____

3. I've been told that I twitch or jerk a lot when I'm asleep.
   True _____ False _____

If you answered "true" to questions 1 and 2, you may be suffering from a condition called Restless Leg Syndrome (RLS). This condition causes unpleasant sensations like tickling, deep aching, or mild to severe muscle spasms in the lower limbs. The discomfort occurs most often just before sleep but also may occur during the sleep period. Stretching, flexing, or repositioning the limb—even getting up and walking—is the only way to get relief. Needless to say, this can upset both your own and your partner's sleep. If question 3 sounds like you, you may have a related condition called Periodic Limb Movement Disorder. EEG readings show that these twitches and movements cause arousal in the brain that increases light sleep and decreases deeper stages.

Strangeness in the Night

You probably won't be surprised to learn that certain abnormal behaviors, such as sleepwalking, bed-wetting, and acting out one's dreams (a condition called REM Behavior Disorder), tend to disrupt sleep. Nightmares and night terrors also upset your ability to get the sleep you need. Answer these questions to find out if you suffer from an abnormal sleep behavior, also known as a *parasomnia*.

Words to Sleep By

A **parasomnia** is any behavioral disturbance that occurs during sleep, such as bed-wetting, sleepwalking or sleeptalking.

1. I've been told that I frequently grind my teeth.
   True _____ False _____

2. I walk in my sleep.
   True _____ False _____

3. I've woken up to find that I've eaten food while I thought I was asleep.
   True _____ False _____

4. I wet the bed.
   True _____ False _____

5. I suffer from nightmares or night terrors.
   True _____ False _____

6. I often awaken feeling confused.
   True _____ False _____

If you answered "true" to any of these questions, you may be suffering from a behavioral sleep disturbance. In Chapter 10, we'll discuss both RLS and the parasomnias in depth and provide you with some tips that will help you help control these behaviors. Like other sleep disorders, however, solving such problems often requires help from medical specialists.

Getting Out of Sync

Remember the information we gave you in Chapter 1 about internal body rhythms? Needless to say, if you're trying to sleep when your body wants to stay up, or vice versa, you're going to run into trouble. See if such a situation applies to you by answering the following statements.

1. I work a night shift or rotating shift.
   True _____ False _____

2. I tend to fall asleep much later than I want to.
   True _____ False _____

3. I regularly fall asleep much earlier than I want to.
   True _____ False _____

4. On weekends and vacations, I go to bed and wake up at significantly different times than I do on my regular schedule.
   True _____ False _____

5. Even on a regular work schedule, I am unable to keep a consistent sleep schedule no matter how hard I try.
   True _____ False _____

If you answered "true" to two or more of these statements, you may be suffering from a circadian rhythm disorder. If so, you'd probably be able to get enough sleep, if only you could sleep when your body prefers to. In Chapter 10, we'll help you make the best of your particular circadian rhythm problem, as well as identify when you might need the help of a sleep specialist.

Is Your Lifestyle Keeping You Up?

Barring any medical problems or special circumstances like night-shift work or time-zone travel, you should be able to get the sleep you need quite naturally. But if you're reading this book, chances are you're failing in this area.

Why? Our best guess is that something in your daily life is disrupting your physiology, preventing your body from easing its way into sleep—thus preventing the body and brain from recovering and renewing themselves before facing the next day's challenges.

To find out what in your day-to-day life is getting in the way of a good night's sleep, take the following quiz.

The Influence of Lifestyle Quiz

Part A: Lifestyle Habits

Answer "Yes" or "No" to the following statements.

1. I am at least 20 pounds overweight.

   Yes _____ No _____

2. I frequently eat dinner within two hours of bedtime.

   Yes _____ No _____

3. I frequently drink caffeinated beverages, often after 6 p.m.

   Yes _____ No _____

4. I lead a sedentary life.

   Yes _____ No _____

5. Most of my exercise periods occur within two hours of bedtime.

   Yes _____ No _____

If you answered "yes" to even one of these questions, you may be able to trace your sleep problem to your diet or exercise habits. You'll find more information about these aspects of sleep hygiene in Chapter 5.

Part B: The Impact of Stress

Answer the following statements 1) Usually, 2) Sometimes, or 3) Rarely.

1. I end the day feeling unsatisfied with my accomplishments. ____

2. During the day, I don't feel I have much control over my work and personal life. ____

3. I don't practice yoga, meditation, or other relaxation strategy. ____

4. I worry about getting to sleep. ____

5. I'm unable to shut out thoughts about responsibilities, unfinished business, or other worries during the evening and night. ____

If you often answered with "usually," you need to find a way to reduce the amount of stress and tension you feel on a day-to-day basis. We'll help you do just that in Chapter 5.

Part C: Appreciating Proper Sleep Hygiene

Answer "Yes" or "No" to the following statements.

1. I watch television or do paperwork in bed before sleep.

    Yes ____ No ____

2. My mattress is more than 5 years old and sags.

    Yes ____ No ____

3. Noise and light have easy access into my bedroom.

    Yes ____ No ____

4. I suffer from allergies and haven't taken steps to remove my allergy triggers from my bedroom.

   Yes _____ No _____

5. I rarely go to bed at the same time or follow the same routine before bed.

   Yes _____ No _____

You've probably already guessed that if you answered "yes" to one or more questions in this quiz, your bedroom may have become your worst enemy when it comes to sleep. In Chapter 6, we'll show you how to create a sleep-enhancing bedroom—starting with the bed and working around the room.

Part D: The Pharmaceutical Industry

Answer "Yes" or "No" to the following statements.

1. I take prescription sleeping pills on many or most nights.

   Yes _____ No _____

2. I use over-the-counter sleep remedies more than once a week.

   Yes _____ No _____

3. If I don't use medication, I cannot sleep well.

   Yes _____ No _____

4. I use herbal potions and teas to help me relax.

   Yes _____ No _____

5. I take melatonin supplements on a regular basis.

   Yes _____ No _____

If you answered "yes" to even one of these questions, you must pay special attention to Chapter 7, where we'll discuss natural and artificial sleep remedies and supplements. Prescription and over-the-counter sleep remedies have a definite and useful purpose when it comes to solving sleep problems, but they must be used with great care and often under a doctor's watchful eye.

Part E: The Power of Light

Answer "Yes" or "No" to the following statements.

1. I rarely get outside in the sunlight during the day.

   Yes _____ No _____

2. My office has no windows that let in sunlight.

   Yes _____ No _____

3. My energy level diminishes during the fall and winter.

   Yes _____ No _____

4. If I get up and outside in the light early in the morning, I go to sleep earlier at night.

   Yes _____ No _____

5. My bedroom never gets completely dark.

   Yes _____ No _____

Did you answer even one question with a "yes"? Since the natural rise and fall of the sun is our primary Zeitgeber, it's no wonder we have such difficulty attaining regular, good sleep. In Chapter 6, we'll show you how light can become your best friend in your quest for a good night's sleep.

Part F: To Nap or Not to Nap

Answer the following statements 1) Usually, 2) Sometimes, or 3) Rarely.

1. I feel sleepy but am unable to sleep during the day.
   _____

2. When I nap, it is typically for longer than 30 minutes but less than one and a-half hours. _____

3. I nap after I get home from work, around 6 p.m.
   _____

4. I don't have the time and place to nap at work.
   _____

5. I wake up from a nap feeling paralyzed and groggy.
   _____

How many questions provoked a "Usually" response from you? The more 1's you wrote down, the more likely it is that you've never made napping a successful part of your sleep pattern—which would be just fine if you were also sleeping well during the night. Since you're having trouble, however, we'll show you in Chapter 8 how a daytime nap can help you get the sleep you need.

In the next several chapters, we'll outline some healthy habits that will help you get a better night's sleep. If you have a particular problem you've identified—say with exercise or stress reduction—feel free to skip to the chapter that you feel most applies to you. We suggest, though, that you read straight through. You're sure to find useful and interesting information in every chapter. We'll start by creating an eating and exercise plan designed to optimize your sleep.

Chapter 5

Healthy Body, Healthy Sleep

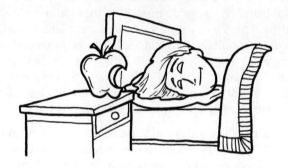

In This Chapter

➤ Understanding the effect of daily habits on sleep

➤ Exploring the effects of food on sleep

➤ Reducing stress

➤ Learning about the sleep-inducing power of exercise

Eating a balanced diet, exercising on a regular basis, reducing toxic levels of stress. . .this triumvirate of good habits is one that few Americans uphold, which may be at least part of the reason that sleep problems are so prevalent. Unfortunately, in addition to messing with your waistline and threatening your health in myriad ways, a failure to establish healthy eating, exercise, and stress-reduction patterns can also affect your ability to sleep well. The good news is that by making certain regular changes in these areas of your daily life, you significantly increase your chances of sleeping well. In this chapter, we'll show you how.

The Diet Connection

Although it's probably not the first thing you think of when identifying risk factors for insomnia, your diet does indeed influence the way you sleep. First, healthy people generally enjoy healthy sleep—or at least they stand a much better chance of doing so than those who are less healthy. That's why eating a balanced diet that includes lots of fresh fruits and vegetables, low levels of fat and sugar, and plenty of variety will help you improve your sleep. This same diet will also help you maintain a healthy weight, which in turn reduces your risk for the sleep disorder Obstructive Sleep Apnea, discussed in Chapter 9.

In addition, the choices you make about how much and what kinds of food you eat in the hours before bedtime have a direct impact on how well you're able to sleep that night. After all, when you think about it, food is made up of chemicals that can act on the body the same way a drug might work. Eating certain foods can help you sleep better by boosting levels of natural sleep-promoting substances in your body. Eating other foods may prevent you from sleeping well by disrupting the function of your brain's sleep centers. Read on for more information.

Rest Easy

Developing a relatively set schedule for your mealtimes, exercise sessions, and other routine day-to-day activities will help you in your quest for regular, restful sleep. Your body runs on an internal clock, and the more you make use of external Zeitgebers, the more likely you'll be to maintain a healthy sleep/wake pattern.

Food for Sleep

Hungry for a late night snack? Well, if you have trouble sleeping, you may be able to help alleviate the problem by making more careful choices when you're choosing your munchies.

Optimally, you want to choose foods that contain the amino acid tryptophan. Tryptophan is important for sleep because it is the precursor of the neurotransmitter called *serotonin,* one of the body's "sleep" chemicals (and a primary neurotransmitter involved in regulating your moods). One of the functions of serotonin is to slow down nerve activity, therefore inducing sleep. Tryptophan is also the precursor of melatonin, the "sleep hormone" that helps set the stage for sleep.

Words to Sleep By

Serotonin is a neurotransmitter, or chemical messenger, important in a wide variety of brain functions, including the regulation of moods. People who suffer from depression, as well as depression-related insomnia, often have deficient levels of serotonin in the brain.

A glass of warm milk contains tryptophan—that's why it's often prescribed as a sleep aid (unless you're lactose-intolerant and the resulting upset stomach would keep you awake). Other foods high in tryptophan include peanut butter, dates, figs, rice, tuna, turkey (which is one of the reasons you get sleepy after Thanksgiving dinner!), and yogurt. It takes about an hour for tryptophan to reach the brain after you consume it, so plan your snacktime wisely. It's also possible to take tryptophan in the form of a supplement, a fact discussed at more length in Chapter 7.

In addition to timing the consumption of tryptophan-rich foods, you may also want to look at whether you're receiving enough vitamins and minerals in your regular diet. Certain vitamins and minerals affect your ability to sleep and the quality of the sleep you get, including vitamin B complex, calcium and magnesium (taken together), copper and iron, and zinc. However, you should discuss taking these substances with a health care professional before using them to help you sleep.

Set Your Alarm!

Take vitamins and supplements with care. Check with your doctor before taking more than the minimum daily requirement of any mineral or vitamin.

As you can see, the substances you put—or fail to put—into your body may influence your ability to sleep. However, if you decide to take supplements or change your diet, you might want to add a category to your Sleep Log that tracks the changes you make and the effects they have. Make one change at a time, then write down its effect, if any, on your sleep over the next few weeks.

Perhaps the biggest concern when it comes to diet and sleep has nothing to do with the food you eat, but rather with the beverages you drink. Indeed, two common substances found in popular drinks—caffeine and alcohol—are major, but avoidable, sleep bandits. (As we'll discuss later, caffeine is found not only in coffee, tea, and cola, but also in many foods.)

The Caffeine Buzz

In the United States alone, more than 80 percent of adults consume caffeine on a regular basis and, on average, ingest the caffeine equivalent of about three cups of coffee a day (about 280 milligrams). A select few of us (about 20 percent) have really got it bad, consuming up to 500 mg or more.

As ubiquitous as caffeine is, it's a drug that produces intense effects on the human mind and body. For most people, the effects are pleasurable. But for others, just a little bit of caffeine on a regular basis can lead to fragmented concentration, headaches, heartburn, irritability, shakiness, chronic gastrointestinal problems, and—yes indeed—insomnia.

As you may already know, caffeine is a stimulant, a member of a group of alkaloids called xanthine derivatives. Within 15 minutes of consuming caffeine, the drug begins to take effect. It acts to increase the amount of the hormone epinephrine (also known as adrenaline) and triggers the following biological events:

➤ An increase of heart rate and blood pressure

➤ An increase in respiration rate (because caffeine also relaxes smooth muscle tissues such as those that line the bronchial tubes)

➤ An increase in the production of stomach acid

➤ An increase in urinary output

➤ Stimulation of brain activity

The effect caffeine produces varies considerably from person to person—and that's where it gets tricky. People who are very sensitive to caffeine may find that *any* amount of the substance consumed at *any* point during the day can disrupt sleep. Others find that if they restrict their intake to the early part of the day, and certainly before dinner, they're okay. Virtually all caffeine is eliminated from the body 12 to 24 hours after it was last consumed, taking with it all its effects and side effects.

Reducing the amount of caffeine you drink may be the key to improving your sleep quantity and quality. But doing so isn't always easy. If you're a big coffee or caffeinated-soda drinker, the biggest obstacles that you face are the withdrawal symptoms that often occur when you cut back your daily consumption of caffeine from the amount your body has come to expect. When your body doesn't get what it needs to start its engine, you're liable to suffer headaches, drowsiness, irritability, depression, and other unpleasant symptoms.

The best way to avoid experiencing these symptoms is to slowly cut back on your caffeine consumption, using less and less every day. The following tips will help you get started:

➤ **Keep track.** Once you figure out how much caffeine you consume and decide to cut back, keep track of the effects of reduced consumption in your daily Sleep Log. In addition, check the labels on the foods, beverages, and medications you consume for the amount of caffeine they contain.

➤ **Take your time.** If you'd like to reduce the amount of caffeine you drink—or eliminate it from your diet altogether—it's best to do so slowly and spread it out over time by reducing the amount you consume by 20 percent each week. For example, if you drink five cups of coffee a day, cut back by just one cup a day the first week, then another cup the next week, and so on until you start to feel better.

The Pitfalls of Alcohol

A brandy before bedtime is one of the oldest prescriptions for a good night's sleep. Unfortunately, drinking alcohol anywhere close to bedtime may disturb rather than aid sleep.

While alcohol may help you fall asleep faster, it can significantly diminish the quality of sleep you obtain during the night. For example, having alcohol in your system can cause you to wake up prematurely—sometimes with an urgent need to urinate. It can also reduce the time you spend in REM sleep (see Chapter 2). Drinking too much alcohol at bedtime is also associated with an increase in snoring and sleep apnea.

However, as is true for caffeine, the effects of alcohol vary considerably among individuals. Many people enjoy a glass of wine or two with dinner and suffer no ill effects. Some even manage quite well having a liqueur or brandy within an hour or two before bedtime. Others, however, are unable to tolerate any alcohol in their systems and, therefore, should avoid it for several hours before they try to sleep.

A second consideration comes into play when it comes to alcohol, and that is dependence. There's quite a difference between enjoying a nightcap before bed and *needing* a nightcap in order to sleep. Once you start to cross over that line, you may need some help in cutting back on the amount of alcohol you drink on a daily basis, or eliminating alcohol altogether.

If you have any questions about how alcohol may be affecting your sleep—or any aspect of your life, for that matter—talk to your doctor about it. In the meantime, it's a good idea for you to carefully track how much you drink and how well you sleep on the nights you drink. If, after a few weeks, you see that you've established an unhealthy pattern, it's time to take control.

One way to start reducing your dependence on alcohol is by looking at the amount of stress in your life: The better you can manage this ubiquitous fact of life, the less likely you'll be to need, rather than simply enjoy, that glass of wine or brandy before bed.

The Perils of Stress

Although we use the word stress often, it isn't always easy to define stress or how it makes you feel. One reason is because, except in extreme situations like the death of a loved one or the threat of imminent physical harm, a clear definition of stress is not available.

Everything that occurs in your life or exists in your environment is technically a stressor because it causes some internal change. If it is very hot out, for example, your body will adjust to the increased ambient temperature by increasing heat loss through the skin by redirecting blood flow toward the skin surface and by cooling the skin with perspiration. In this instance, heat is a stressor because it poses a challenge that spurs the body to action. In addition, stressors vary in their effect from person to person. For some, a day spent lying on a beach is completely relaxing; for others such forced recreation is sheer torture. Again, it's how you as an individual *perceive* a situation that determines how your body reacts to it.

Rest Easy

If you find yourself having to leave the bedroom at night because of insomnia, find a comfortable spot in which to set yourself and choose a relaxing activity (like reading or knitting) rather than something stimulating (like doing your bills!). It is crucial, however, that you go back to bed only when you start to feel very sleepy, and not before.

Despite the difficulties in defining and measuring stress, there is no doubt that a strong connection exists between the mind, the emotions, and all aspects of health, including how well we sleep. Before we continue this discussion of the impact of stress on sleep, let's see just what happens to the body when faced with a stressful situation.

Understanding Stress

Whether you're conscious of it or not, your body has a remarkable gift for self-preservation. When its internal balance is threatened in any way, it mobilizes immediately, preparing you either to battle the impending danger or to flee from it. We call this the "fight-or-flight response," and we're probably more used to thinking about it as occurring during times of physical danger. Let's say that seemingly out of nowhere, a bus bears down on you while you're crossing the street. Your heart starts to pound and the muscles in your legs and arms tense up. Before you know it, you're across the street, running faster and harder than you'd ever thought possible. However, even low levels of stress can mean that your heart beats just a little too fast and your muscles tense up just a little too much for you to fall and stay asleep.

Set Your Alarm!

Don't take signs that your body and mind are overloaded with stress lightly. Among the signs of stress are chronic muscle aches, gastrointestinal distress, and—yes!—insomnia. See your doctor: Stress is implicated in a host of life-threatening diseases, including heart disease, high blood pressure, and stroke.

In addition, the more stress you feel, the more likely you are to engage in other behaviors detrimental to both your general health and your ability to get a good night's sleep, namely drinking alcohol, smoking cigarettes, overeating, and failing to exercise.

Later in this chapter, you'll learn new strategies for relieving stress in your life that emphasize bringing healthy, positive energy into your life and your body through meditation and relaxation. But first, let's see if you can evaluate just how stressed out you really are, and how that may be affecting your ability to sleep.

Identifying Your Stress Triggers

You've just read about the powerful impact stress has on the body and how that can influence your general health and your sleep patterns. Now we suggest that you take the time to track your reactions to everyday stressful occurrences. How do you feel when your train is late? Or when a bill you thought had been paid turns up overdue? We've devised a daily Stress Log that might help you identify the source of your stress and track not only your immediate reaction to the situation but also the end result. We're betting that at the end of the week, you'll discover that one way you can reduce stress is by first recognizing, and then letting go of, things you can't control—things that usually do not disrupt your life in any significant or long-lasting ways.

We suggest that you track your stress triggers and responses. Simply write down what stresses you out, what time the stressor occurred, how it made you feel, and what you can do next time to avoid reacting in the same negative and ultimately undermining way.

Once you've found out what really bugs you during the day, your next task is to learn to reduce any resulting stress. Needless to say, one of the most effective ways of reducing stress is to eliminate as many stress-causing agents from your life as possible: changing from your present job to one less fraught with tension, moving to a place more suited to your personality and taste, avoiding people who annoy you, and so on. Unfortunately, making such changes often is easier said than done; they'll take some long-range planning and, no doubt, a good deal of self-examination. Not a bad idea, but maybe not so practical when you already can't think straight for lack of sleep!

Reducing Stress: Two Easy Exercises

This is a simple meditation exercise that can help you relax and focus your attention away from the things that cause stress in your life. Start by sitting for just 5 to 10 minutes until you feel comfortable with the practice, then work up to 30 minutes. You may find it helpful to perform your meditation just before going to sleep, but anytime you do it will help reduce overall stress levels. In fact, until you've begun to solve your sleep problem, you may want to avoid practicing this strategy at bedtime when the stakes for relaxing are so high and tension may be the result of a "failed" attempt at meditation.

Basic Meditation Exercise

1. Wear loose, comfortable clothing.

2. Find a quiet place where you won't be disturbed. Turn off the TV or radio, unplug the phone, and ask your family and pets for some privacy.

3. Sit on the floor or bed in a comfortable position. Allow your hands to rest on your legs.

4. Lower your gaze so that your eyes are almost, but not quite, closed.

5. Take a deep breath and let it out slowly.

6. The easiest way to begin meditation is to count your breaths. Inhale, count one. Exhale, count two. Inhale, count three. Repeat the process until you exhale at number ten. Start again, with an inhale, count one.

Another approach to relaxation—and one that's perfect to do in bed as you try to sleep—is deep breathing. When you become distressed, your breathing becomes rapid and shallow. When you're more relaxed, on the other hand, you're probably breathing more slowly and regularly.

Deep Breathing Exercise

1. Get into bed, turn off the lights, and lie flat on your back in a comfortable position.

2. Close your eyes and attempt to concentrate on just your breathing. Leave behind the worries or joys of your day and think only of this moment in time.

3. Visualize your breathing system as consisting of three parts—your abdomen, the middle part near your diaphragm (just beneath your rib cage), and the upper space in your chest. (Please note that only your lungs actually fill with air, but this imagery may help you learn to take deeper, fuller breaths.)

4. As you breathe in through your nose, picture the lower space filling first. Allow your abdomen to expand as air enters the space. Then visualize your middle space filling with energy, light, and air and feel your waistline expand. Feel your chest and your upper back open up as air continues to fill the lungs. The inhalation should take about five seconds.

5. When your lungs feel comfortably full, stop the intake of air.

6. Exhale in a controlled, smooth, continuous movement, the air streaming steadily out of the nostrils. Feel your chest, middle, and stomach gently contract.

Continue to breathe in this way, concentrating only on your breath. With each inhalation, take in serenity and peace. With each exhalation, let go of worry and physical tension. Before you know it, you'll be asleep.

Work It Out

The benefits of regular exercise are almost too numerous to mention. In addition to reducing your risk of developing heart disease, high blood pressure, some kinds of cancer, and many other diseases, exercise helps improve your mood and reduce stress. As a wonderful side effect, it also improves the quality of your sleep.

The Sleep-Promoting Benefits of Exercise

Contrary to popular belief, exercise doesn't help you sleep by making your body tired. People who have trouble sleeping aren't helped even when they are physically exhausted. Instead, exercise alleviates physical stress and certain medical disorders that may affect sleep. Here are just a few of the reasons you might want to add exercise to your life if you're having trouble getting a good night's sleep:

➤ **Exercise helps you fall asleep faster.** In one recent study, a regular exercise routine cut the time it took to fall asleep in half—from 28 to 14 minutes. The study focused on a group of formerly sedentary people who had completed a 16-week program of moderate exercise.

➤ **Exercise helps you sleep longer.** The same study found that exercise added an average of more than 45 minutes to the participants' main sleep blocks.

➤ **Exercise improves sleep quality.** To wake up feeling refreshed, you need to spend a good proportion of your time in bed in deep sleep. A 1994 study found that people who completed an aerobic training course experienced a 33 percent increase in sleep Stages 3 and 4—the slow-wave sleep that is the deepest type of sleep.

➤ **Exercise at certain times can help shift your biological clock.** Recent research suggests that exercise offers a bonus for people who must be up at night, either for work or for personal obligations. It shifts circadian rhythms, indirectly leading to a better mood and alertness on the work schedule or shift you choose to follow. In Chapters 11 and 12, on time-zone travel and night work, we'll discuss this subject in more depth.

Making Exercise a Part of Your Life

If you're sedentary, making exercise a regular part of your life will take a little work, a lot of commitment, and some perseverance. The benefits, though, will be well worth the effort: You'll not only improve your overall health, you may just improve the quality of your sleep.

When it comes to exercising in order to increase your chances of getting a good night's sleep, it's best to focus on increasing the amount of cardiovascular exercise you get. That means walking, running, playing singles tennis, swimming, and bicycling, to name just a few activities. At the same time, if you prefer yoga and weight-training, by all means, start there. Whatever you do to increase your physical fitness and help yourself relieve stress will improve the quality and quantity of sleep you obtain.

Here are a few tips to get you started:

➤ **Start slowly.** Don't overdo. If you try to put in two hours a day every day during your first week exercising, you'll only end up sore and discouraged—and *very* unlikely to want to work out the next week. The best way to stick to exercising is to start small and build gradually: 20 to 30 minutes are all you need to start improving your level of fitness.

➤ **Time exercise sessions with care.** If getting to sleep at night is difficult for you, try exercising in the late afternoon or early evening. Exercise helps raise the body temperature, helping set the stage for sleep. DO NOT exercise within 3 hours of bedtime, however. You'll only stimulate your muscles and increase your alertness, making it more difficult than ever for you to fall asleep. Some people find exercising in the late afternoon is best, since muscular performance is best and tolerance for physical stress appears to be highest at this time.

Rest Easy

If you're an extreme Owl, getting your exercise outside in the sunlight early in the day can help shift your biological clock forward, so that you'll get up a little earlier in the day and go to bed a little earlier at night—and feel better doing it!

➤ **Set realistic goals.** If you've been sedentary for a number of months or years, deciding to train for next month's marathon by running 10 miles every morning would be counterproductive and even dangerous to your health. Instead, set goals just barely within your reach. Achieving them will give you a sense of pride and self-confidence that's sure to keep you motivated.

➤ **Add variety.** To alleviate boredom, try alternating activities. Take a dance class one session, bicycle outside the next, or perform yoga postures every other morning. By varying your routine, you're more likely to keep it going.

Timing Is Everything

It's never too late to make positive changes in your life. If you're having trouble falling or staying asleep, now is the time to look at the ways your daily diet, stress levels, and exercise habits might be keeping you up at night. Next, we'll take you into your bedroom to see how your sleep environment can help or hinder your efforts to obtain sufficient shut-eye.

Chapter 6

Setting the Stage for Sleep

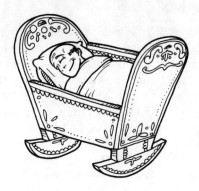

In This Chapter

➤ Understanding the importance of a proper sleep environment

➤ Examining your bedroom with sleep in mind

➤ Accounting for light—at night and throughout the year

➤ Establishing a healthy pre-sleep routine

There's a time and place for everything, as the expression goes—and when it comes to sleep, it's especially true. As this chapter will explain, creating an environment conducive for sleep and developing a regular routine for bedtime may help you solve your current sleep problem. First you'll read about the factors in your sleep environment that may be adversely affecting you, then you'll take a quiz that will help you rate the quality of your current sleep environment. We'll also give you plenty of tips to create a healthy, sleep-promoting haven for yourself.

Creating Your Sanctuary

Ironically enough, the bedroom is often the last place we think to look when searching for a reason for our sleep difficulties. But that's exactly where at least part of the problem may lie.

Take a good look at your bedroom now. Is it free of clutter and distraction? Or is sleeping only one of the many things you do in this room? Does it have window shades that keep out the light? How noisy is it during the night? Is it a "safe zone" in which you can expect a certain amount of privacy and freedom from interruption during your naps and major sleep periods? Let's just see.

Clearing the Distractions

It makes sense, doesn't it, that you'd want the room that you sleep in to have a sense of calmness about it, to be free from the ordinary stresses and strains of the day? But if you're like most people, you've got your television plugged in near your bed, your laptop computer on a nearby desk, and the mail piled up on the nightstand. If that sounds like your room, your first priority is to clear away as much of that clutter as you can. Having a serene environment for sleep is one of the first rules of proper sleep hygiene.

In most cases, the first thing you should banish from the bedroom is the television set. While some people find that watching a little television helps put them to sleep, many others—especially those already having difficulty falling asleep—are actually quite stimulated by it. Its frantic images, its too-loud commercials, its often anxiety-inducing news reports, and the simple space it takes up in your mind make television an unlikely candidate for the world's most relaxing activity.

If you find yourself awake and watching television far later than you'd like, then put the set into another room.

Watch it there until you feel sleepy, then go back to your bedroom for sleep. Moving the TV out of your bedroom also means that you'll be much less likely to turn it on and then become distracted by it if you awaken in the middle of the night.

Rest Easy

If you live in a studio apartment, or otherwise simply have no way to separate your work/living space from your sleep space, consider purchasing one or two inexpensive folding screens to place around the potential source of distraction.

As is true for so many sleep solutions, however, you may have to experiment a bit to see if television is a help or a hindrance to your sleep. If you've got a routine that works for you—if hearing Jay Leno's monologue is your sure-fire cue that it's bedtime—then don't mess with it. If not, and you suspect your insomnia may be due to, or exacerbated by, watching too many late, late movies, then remove temptation by removing the television set.

Of course, the TV isn't the only potential source of distraction in your bedroom. Your home computer, a stack of mail, or even just the presence of your briefcase can trigger thoughts of work, bills, and other responsibilities. If you can, clear your nightstand of all but a bedside lamp, an alarm clock (maybe), and perhaps a pleasant vase of your favorite flowers. (We'll get to the issue of clocks in the bedroom a bit later!)

Hush, Hush

It's also important to monitor your bedroom for sounds that could be disrupting your sleep. If you find that you're exposed to the sound of noisy neighbors, air or street traffic, or other noise while in your bedroom, try using earplugs to shut out all sound. You may also find it helpful to try "white noise"—the sound of an air-conditioner in the summertime, for instance, or the static of a radio set between two stations. You can also try one of the new "environmental sound" machines that play the sounds of the surf or the rain. Many people find these sounds block out disturbing noises and help relax them so they get to sleep.

Set Your Alarm!

Hide and mute that tick-tock. If you're like most people with insomnia, any reminder of the passage of time is a source of stress and anxiety. Put your alarm clock—preferably a digital one that runs silently and is illuminated—inside a dresser drawer. If you'll only become more stressed if you don't have access to the clock, at least turn the clock face from view.

Another factor in your sleep environment is light. Too much light at night can thwart even your best efforts to establish a healthy sleep pattern, while light at the right time can help you reset your body clock so that you can sleep when you need to.

The Light That's Right

If you're like most people, you'll sleep best when it's completely dark in your bedroom. Make sure the hall and bathroom lights are off (or shut the door against them) and cover all windows that get morning light, or light from street lamps and passing cars. Window shades and lined drapes (or a combination of both) are often sufficient for this purpose, but if you're especially sensitive to incoming light, you may want to purchase special blackout shades that totally cover the window surface. Another alternative is wearing eye shades, which are effective in blocking out the light.

It's important to understand that even the light from a street lamp can disturb your ability to fall or stay asleep—if it's shining directly in your window. You may not even realize how greatly you're disturbed by excess light in the bedroom until you take the time to assess just how much light streams in from the hallway, bathroom, or outside. Tonight, turn off the lights, allow your eyes to adjust to the darkness, and evaluate how dark (or light) your bedroom really is.

In addition to this aspect of light/dark and sleep, it's important for you to understand just how important our primary Zeitgeber really is when it comes to sleep and other daily cycles. The path of sunlight across the surface of our spinning planet, with its regular progression of sunrises and sunsets, and our planet's revolution around the sun determined much of our ancestors' day-to-day and seasonal lives, from when they got up in the morning to when they planted their crops. These days, most of us frequently become disconnected from the natural rhythms set by the sun, which could be one reason why so many people have sleep problems.

Most people in modern, industrial societies receive too much of the wrong kind of light (primarily dim, artificial light) and too little of the right kind (full-spectrum bright natural daylight). Because of this, we inadvertently play havoc with our internal circadian clocks, thereby disrupting our sleep, our moods, and other aspects of our physical and mental health.

Learning about the potential effects of light on your sleep/
wake patterns will help you better manipulate your exposure to it in order to improve your sleep at night and alertness levels during the day. In this chapter, we'll show you
how to do just that.

Light and Your Brain

The intensity of the light falling on us is measured in *lux,*
which is the international unit of illumination. When
you're standing outside, you're exposed to about 10,000
lux on a heavy, overcast day, 50,000 lux on a sunny day,
and 100,000 lux or more on an open beach or snow-
covered ground where much light is reflected from the
surface. By contrast, indoor light from incandescent or
fluorescent light bulbs may provide only 200 to 500 lux,
depending on how far you are from the light source.
Many industrial workplaces provide even less light at
night. In such places, light levels of 5 to 50 lux—or even
less—are common. People who work at computer stations
controlling oil refineries or nuclear power stations, for instance, may receive less than 5 lux.

Words to Sleep By

Lux is the metric unit used to quantify the intensity of
visible light. It represents the amount of light that eventually falls upon an object or a person from a source—not
necessarily the amount of light being emitted from that
source.

The primary way the brain receives light is through the
eyes, though recent research indicates that other body
cells (including, perhaps, blood cells) are also sensitive to
light. Light sends a signal that is conveyed to that tiny

group of brain cells called the suprachiasmatic nuclei (SCN). As we mentioned earlier, these cells appear to be the master internal clock that drives the body's sleep/wake and other biological patterns. As discussed in Chapter 1, light in the morning and darkness at night are the two most important cues that keep these rhythms in synch. Without regular and well-timed exposure to the natural cycles of light and darkness, you may well end up with a sleep problem.

Understanding the Timing of Light

When it comes to how light affects your biological rhythms, you must consider not only how bright the light is, but also when you're exposed to it. Indeed, the effect that light has on your circadian rhythms depends to a large degree on what time of day or night you are exposed to it.

As we've discussed, light is the primary Zeitgeber, the cue that helps maintain your daily rhythms by signaling the time of day to the brain. Therefore, depending on what point in the day or night exposure to bright light occurs, you can either advance or delay your circadian rhythms. Your body clock's reaction to light falls on a continuum, called the phase response curve (PRC). The PRC describes the number of hours of shift in the setting of the biological clock that occurs when an individual is exposed to bright light.

Rest Easy

If you have trouble getting to sleep at night, try turning off all but the most necessary lights in your home—even relatively dim light bulbs can have a stimulating effect on your body.

During the day, your biological clock virtually ignores light signals, since that's when it naturally expects sunlight to fall. At night, between the hours of 10 p.m. and 5 a.m., however, exposure to sufficiently bright light acts to delay the timing of the clock, in effect shifting it westward. The later and the more intense this exposure is, the greater the shift westward. Exposure to light from 5 a.m. to 8 a.m., on the other hand, nudges the biological clock eastward. The strongest shifts westward or eastward occur when exposure to light takes place closest to the "breakpoint" of about 5 a.m., or about two hours before normal wake-up time, which is near your body temperature minimum.

Let's say you're jetting off from Boston to Paris and want to know how to best avoid jet lag by resetting your clock. When do you need exposure to light? If you're like most travelers, you'll get off the plane at 7 a.m. local time—but at 1 a.m. body time. Light in the early Paris morning will reset your clock westward toward Hawaii time—in the totally wrong direction. Instead of taking a stroll outside, keep your sunglasses on until you reach your hotel, stay in the darkness (napping if you like) until about 11 a.m., then go outside and sit in the sun. A precisely timed exposure to the light from 11 a.m. to 1 p.m. will help you adapt to the local scene much more quickly than you otherwise would. We'll discuss this further in Chapter 11.

Providing light in the right amounts at the right time to help you solve your sleep problems—whether they're caused by a sleep disorder, time-zone travel, or night-shift work—is tricky business, one better left to sleep specialists. However, you can see that bright light exposure is an important factor in your sleep/wake patterns. Depending on your climate, or on your individual needs, finding the right light may be a challenge.

When Light Interferes with Health

In addition to helping set and maintain your body's internal clock, light also enhances your alertness. Both bright and moderate light cause you to become more awake and alert than you might otherwise be. In laboratory studies at the Institute for Circadian Physiology, for instance, people who were exposed to 1,000 lux during simulated night shifts were less likely to fall asleep on the job, and they also scored better on cognitive performance tests than workers left in the relative dark.

Exactly why light enhances alertness is not well understood. The leading theory is that light suppresses the brain's production of melatonin, a hormone that promotes sleepiness. Some studies also indicate that exposure to light raises body temperature, which helps boost alertness and mental performance.

As you can see, light significantly affects when you wake, when you sleep, and how you feel—a point we'll discuss further in later chapters. In addition, certain individuals are quite dramatically affected by the loss of light during the fall and winter months, developing a clinical syndrome known as Seasonal Affective Disorder (SAD).

People with SAD suffer from most of the usual symptoms of depression—sadness, helplessness, hopelessness, guilt, and mild illness—but also have other symptoms specific to this disorder. They tend to eat more rather than less during this time, experience weight gain, and crave rich carbohydrates. They spend many more hours than usual asleep, yet feel chronically exhausted and lethargic. Researchers now believe that the problem in people with SAD is that they are highly sensitive to the changes in day length that occur during the autumn and winter, and that their biological rhythms fall out of synch as a result.

Two sleep disorders called Advanced Sleep Phase Syndrome (ASPS) and Delayed Sleep Phase Syndrome (DSPS) are alsorelated to the effects of light on the biological clock. People who suffer from ASPS become sleepy very early in the evening and wake up very early in the morning. When left to their own devices, those with Delayed Sleep Phase Disorder get up very late in the morning and cannot fall asleep until the wee hours just before dawn. On vacations or weekends, both groups sleep well, once they get to sleep, but do so out of synch with the rest of the world. The problem comes when they try to conform to normal business hours. Researchers believe that those who suffer from ASPS or DSPS may lack a sensitivity to light that would otherwise naturally reset their body clocks and keep them in synch. We'll discuss these disorders in more depth in Chapter 10.

Switching It On. . .and Off

Usually, the best way to get all the bright light you need is to go outside in the sunlight. However, if you suffer from SAD or ASPS/DSPS, or if you live in a climate that doesn't offer enough sun throughout the year, this may not be possible for you. Indeed, people who live in regions with long, dark winters or excessively overcast climates may have more difficulty maintaining their natural sleep/wake cycle, and they also run a greater risk of developing SAD. Other people who could benefit from the right light at the right time are those who work the night shift or travel across time zones and want to avoid exhaustion and jet lag.

Rest Easy

Don't forget that exposure to morning light can help reset your internal biological clock. If you're an extreme Owl, but you want or need to start getting up and going to bed earlier, then allowing the sun to wake you in the morning may be very helpful.

The good news is that technology has come to the rescue once again. In recent years, several companies have developed light boxes and other products to provide bright, full-spectrum light in the home. Prices for these devices range from as little as $300 to as much as $1,000 or more for larger systems. The most efficient ones have special high-intensity fluorescent tubes that use just 150 watts of electricity (and thus cost less than a penny a day to run).

Some light boxes include dusk/dawn lighting controls that simulate natural spring/summer light cycles. You can also get one that you program yourself so that you can simulate (or enhance) sunrise in the morning and darkness falling at night in your bedroom. This way it is possible to awaken from Stage 2 or REM sleep when one will feel most refreshed.

Please note, however, that there are risks and side effects to the use of light boxes, and it's important to talk to your doctor before you try to treat your sleep problem with light therapy. Should you decide upon that course of treatment, follow your doctor's suggestions as well as the instructions that come with the device in order to avoid negative effects, such as headaches, irritability, and eye strain.

Okay, you've got your bedroom in good shape by clearing away distractions, and you understand better how to make light work for instead of against you. Now, let's move on to another aspect of sleep hygiene: the appropriate size and quality of your bed and pillows.

Sleep Like a Log, Not on One!

Take a moment and fantasize about getting into the "perfect bed." Imagine the feeling that you'll get when you slide between crisp, clean sheets onto a firm but giving mattress, then place your head on a soft pillow that provides you with just the right amount of head and neck support. And then. . .and then. . .just fall into a restful, comfortable sleep.

Now go and get into *your* bed. Does reality match up to the fantasy? Or could your bed and its trappings stand some improvement? Needless to say, if you can't get comfortable in bed, you're going to have a lot more trouble falling asleep.

Finding the Right Mattress

If you're one of the vast majority of Americans who own an innerspring mattress, the first question you need to ask yourself when evaluating your current mattress is "Did I buy this before or after Nixon resigned?" Actually, if the answer to that question could even conceivably be "before," you're *way* overdue for a change. The truth is, most mattresses have an average life span of about 10 to 12 years. If you've hit or passed the decade mark, it's time to start thinking about a replacement.

Set Your Alarm!

If you suffer from allergies, be sure to identify and remove potential allergens from the bedroom. Choose bedclothes and pillows with care, remove all rugs (which can become depositories for dust mites, pollen, dander, and other airborne allergens), and consider getting an air-conditioner fitted with a special air filter to keep you breathing easily throughout the night.

One way to check the health of your mattress is to go to a department store and lie down on a brand new mattress. See how it feels, then go home and try your own. If you notice that your old mattress dips and sags, or if you feel the pinch of sprung springs, chances are you're due for a new one. If so, get yourself back to the store—this time, ready to buy.

When buying a new mattress, there are several factors to consider:

➤ **Size.** Make sure that your bed is large enough to provide ample sleeping space for you. If you're very tall or large, or if you sleep with a partner, then you should consider buying a queen- or even a king-size mattress and bed frame. A full (double) bed is only 54 by 75 inches. A queen-size bed, in comparison, is 60 by 80 inches, and a California king is 72 by 84 inches.

➤ **Firmness.** How firm the mattress should be is definitely a matter of taste as well as physiology. A mattress should support your lower back and keep your spine in alignment from its base to your head. If you suffer from arthritis or another condition that causes joint or muscle pain, you probably will feel better on a firmer rather than softer mattress.

➤ **Cost.** Generally speaking, the more you pay, the better mattress you'll get. That said, there is a wide range of prices for satisfactory products, starting at the lower end—about $300—and going all the way up to $1,200 and more. The best advice: Spend as much as you can, and your body will thank you for it.

The Truth About Pillows

Believe it or not, your headaccounts for a full 20 percent of your body weight and, therefore, needs to be well supported when you're lying down. Down or feather pillows are usually best because they "give" better than polyester fills, which can be stiff and inflexible.

Your pillow should support the head and neck, keeping them in alignment with the spine—no matter what sleeping position you take. Generally speaking, you'll want a firmer pillow if you sleep on your side, a medium-firm pillow if you sleep on your back, and a soft pillow if you sleep on your stomach.

Which Way Means Comfortable Sleep?

Back sleepers, side sleepers, stomach sleepers, tossers and turners. . .everyone has his or her favorite sleep style. How you sleep best is the position you want to be in—as long as you also feel comfortable during the day. If you sleep on your stomach and wake with lower back pain, you may want to try adjusting to a side position (some people find that stacking pillows in front of and behind them will help them maintain this position). If you sleep on your back and your partner tells you that you snore, a side position may also help solve this problem.

When all is said and done, however, even the best bedroom environment will do nothing to help a very awake, overstimulated person get to sleep. If you find yourself all wound up with no place to go when it's time for bed, then you may need to re-evaluate how you spend your evening hours.

Finishing Touches

The hour or so before you go to bed is extremely important in setting the stage for an easy descent into sleep. You can make this time work for you by following a regular, restful routine. Here are some tips:

➤ **Avoid stimulation.** About an hour before you want to fall asleep, put away the mail, stop writing down your worries, and simply try to relax.

➤ **Heat up.** A warm bath, preferably one scented with an oil like lavender—known for its calming attributes—is another relaxing ritual that helps set the stage for sleep. In addition to soothing body and soul, a warm bath also raises body temperature—and cooling down afterwards is one of the triggers for sleep.

➤ **Stick to the plan.** As we've tried to make clear in this and previous chapters, when it comes to sleeping well the most important thing about your nighttime experience is setting up a routine that works for you—then sticking to it. Your body's internal clock easily becomes disrupted when unexpected changes occur. If sipping a glass of herbal tea while you take a warm bath provides you with a restful night's sleep, then perform that ritual as often as you can and at as regular a time as possible.

After reading this chapter, how would you rate yoursleep environment and bedtime routine? Take this quiz and see.

Your Sleep Hygiene Quiz

Circle the number that best describes your situation.

1. My room is free from loud or sudden noises.

   Poor   **Excellent**
     1   2   3   4   5

2. I sleep in darkness, using window shades or eye covers if necessary.

   Poor   **Excellent**
     1   2   3   4   5

3. My room temperature allows me to sleep well.

   Poor   **Excellent**
     1   2   3   4   5

4. My mattress and pillow are firm enough to support me and soft enough to offer comfort.

Poor   **Excellent**
1   2   3   4   5

5. I have enough fresh air in my bedroom.

Poor   **Excellent**
1   2   3   4   5

6. I perform regular, relaxing activities (e.g., warm bath, easy stretches, etc.) during the hour or two before I go to bed each night.

Poor   **Excellent**
1   2   3   4   5

Score the quiz by adding up the numbers you circled. If your total score is between 25 and 30, you've designed your bedroom well and have established a nighttime ritual that works for you. If you suffer from insomnia and score between 20 and 25, look at the questions you circled with a "2" or "1" and start making changes there. If you score 20 or less, your bedroom definitely needs some work. Take another look at some of the tips we've offered here, and see if you can improve your sleep by touching up your sleep environment.

Chapter 7

Medicines and Herbs: Pros and Cons

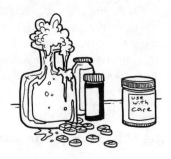

In This Chapter

➤ When sleeping pills and potions might help

➤ The power of narcotics

➤ Understanding the role of melatonin and tryptophan

➤ Exploring herbal remedies

To someone struggling with chronic insomnia, it's often hard to resist the quick-fix approach to getting rid of anxiety and exhaustion so that sleep—deep, restful sleep—is possible. That's why "sleep cures" of all kinds—from prescription medications to over-the-counter remedies to herbal supplements—remain so popular. According to an estimate by the National Sleep Foundation, consumers spend more than $1.1 billion a year on products used to promote sleep.

But like most other ideas that sound too good to be true, these quick fixes usually fail to achieve your ultimate goal—improving your sleep over the long term. By taking any substance to help you sleep, you're treating only the symptom, not the underlying problem. Until you figure out what's really keeping you from getting a good night's sleep, and solving it from that perspective, you'll still have a sleep problem when you wake up the next day.

That said, there is a time and place for such sleep aids. And, if you take them as directed and with care, you may be able to get the rest you need without suffering any adverse effects. In this chapter, we'll help you sort out the myths from the facts about sleeping pills and over-the-counter potions so that you can make a more informed decision about what's right for you.

How Sleeping Pills Work: For and Against You

According to recent research, more than 13 million people in the United States take some kind of prescribed medication to improve their sleep. A sleeping pill is any medication used to promote sleep and treat insomnia. As we'll discuss further in a moment, there are several types of sleeping pills available today, each one affecting the brain and body in a different way.

In general, sleeping pills act to sedate and depress the arousal centers in the brain, thereby promoting sleep (and often reducing anxiety as well). To a greater or lesser degree, depending on their make-up, sleeping pills reduce the time it takes to reach sleep onset and decrease the number of awakenings.

However—and this is a big however—all sleeping pills also have significant drawbacks when it comes to long-term, or even medium-term, use. These drawbacks include:

> ➤ **Sleep quality.** Most sleeping pills alter your sleep architecture, increasing the amount of time you spend in lighter Stage 2 sleep and decreasing the time you

spend in deep Stages 3 and 4 and REM sleep. This means that your brain and body do not receive the full recovery benefits of natural sleep on the nights you take a sleeping aid.

➤ **Dependence.** Taking sleeping pills may create a vicious circle of dependence: Most pills work well only for a relatively short amount of time—a few weeks at most. After that, two things can happen: You not only can become dependent on them, but also may have to up the dosage bit by bit or change medications often in order to reap any benefit. Or you can quit them altogether. In some cases, especially if you only used sleeping pills for a brief period to get yourself through a bad time, you'll be just fine if you quit taking them. If, on the other hand, you're particularly sensitive to the medication, you may develop another problem: *rebound insomnia.*

Words to Sleep By

Rebound insomnia is a common side effect that occurs after sleeping pill use is terminated and the insomnia comes back—sometimes with even more stubbornness than before. REM sleep is also disturbed, and some people report having terrible nightmares.

➤ **Rebound insomnia.** The really miserable thing about overusing sleeping pills is that once you decide to stop, your problem with sleep may only become worse. For reasons not yet completely understood, sudden withdrawal from sleeping pills—sometimes after taking them just a few times—brings back the original insomnia, often with a greater intensity.

And this rebound effect can last up to several weeks. It's best to reduce the dosage slowly.

➤ **Side effects.** Daytime sleepiness, temporary memory loss, confusion, dizziness, weakness, nausea, delayed reaction time, loss of appetite, and frequent urination are some of the many side effects caused by most sleeping pills. Among the most dangerous (as you might suspect) are those that affect your ability to function the next day. Accidents of all kinds are more likely to occur if you are not alert and are unable to react. As is true for the drugs' effects, side effects also vary from individual to individual—some very sensitive people may have strong reactions, while others experience few or no problems at all.

➤ **Risk of interactions.** The active ingredients in sleeping pills can counteract or, conversely, enhance the effects of other medications and alcohol. As central nervous system depressants, they act to slow down respiration and the heart rate, as do alcohol, antihistamines, and some other medications. If you take too much of these central nervous system depressants, the effects can be deadly. Medication used to promote sleep can also interfere with the metabolism of other medications. Therefore, your doctor may need to adjust the dosage appropriately. NEVER DRINK ALCOHOL when you're taking a sleep medication. The result could be lethal.

Prescription Drugs: The Inside Scoop

When choosing a sleeping medication that's right for you, your doctor will take a wide variety of factors into consideration, including your symptoms, what he or she knows about your physiological makeup, other medications you're taking, and the action of the specific drug itself. Among the general choices your doctor has are the following classes of drugs (and within these classes are literally dozens of different medications):

➤ **Benzodiazepines.** Now the most common prescription drugs for insomnia, benzodiazepines induce sleep by suppressing arousal centers in the brain. Compared to older sleeping pills (see below), they have relatively few side effects and drug interactions. Some benzodiazepines (such as triazolam [Halcion]) are short-acting, while others (such as flurazepam [Dalmane]) are long-acting, which can make you feel sleepy during the day. You can become dependent on any of these medications in a relatively short time, however, and they should be used only under the careful direction of a physician.

➤ **Barbiturates.** Barbiturates are sedatives—that is, they act to depress the central nervous system. Not only do they suppress the arousal centers in the brain (helping you sleep), they also affect the heart rate, decrease the blood pressure, and lower body temperature. Because of the wide range of effects and side effects, doctors today almost never prescribe barbiturates to new users, and often advise current users to switch to newer medication. Only in rare cases are barbiturates used to treat insomnia.

➤ **Imidazopyridines.** This new class of drugs, of which only one is now available—under the brand name Ambien (zolpidem)—appears to be far safer than barbiturates and poses even lower risks of side effects, drug interactions, rebound insomnia, and addiction than benzodiazepines. Another benefit of zolpidem is that it does not appear to reduce the time spent in deep and REM sleep stages, one of the biggest drawbacks of some other medications.

➤ **Sedating antidepressants.**Another option for those suffering from insomnia is an antidepressant that also acts as a sedative. Even if you don't also suffer from depression, you might benefit from this treatment if you've experienced side effects from other types of sleeping medication, or have a history of alcohol or drug dependence. Antidepressants also pose little risk of dependence. Unfortunately, they, too, have their potential side effects, including changes in heart rate, dry mouth, urine retention, and impairment in sexual function.

Rest Easy

If you're finding it impossible to sleep because you're facing a particularly difficult emotional or physical challenge, talk to your doctor. Taking a sleeping pill for a few nights may help you regain your strength and prevent insomnia from becoming yet another stressful problem for you to solve.

➤ **Antihistamines.** As anyone who's taken an antihistamine to treat allergies can tell you, this type of medication does more than clear up your sinuses and reduce itching. In most people, certain antihistamines also have a sedating effect that, if timed properly, can help reduce the time it takes to reach sleep onset at night. However, not all antihistamines help to sedate—some actually act as stimulants— and most work only for a night or two at best. Antihistamines can also have significant side effects, including dizziness, gastric distress, dryness of the mouth and nose, and disturbed coordination. You can buy some antihistamines over the counter, while others are by prescription only.

Among the most important qualities of a sleeping medication is its uptake (the time needed for it to take effect) and its *half-life,* (the time needed for your body to break down and eliminate it). Some medications work very quickly, which means you should take them just before or as you go to bed—and these medications may be helpful if middle-of-the-night awakenings are a problem for you. It's also important to know the half-life of a drug because that determines how long the average person will feel its effects—some medications leave your body quickly, whereas others affect you far longer than you might desire. In general, the drugs that have the shortest half-life are your best bets.

Words to Sleep By

The **half-life** of a medication is the length of time it takes for your body to break the drug down into inactive forms or to eliminate it. A drug with a short half-life may be out of your body completely after 5 hours or so, while longer-acting ones may continue to have an effect for 24 hours or more.

Despite the risks of taking medication to help you sleep, we want to state clearly once again that there *are* circumstances that warrant it. The most important thing you can do for your health is to discuss the matter thoroughly with your doctor before taking any medication for this purpose.

You and Your Doctor

Insomnia is one of those symptoms for which there is no objective clinical evidence. That means that your doctor must depend on your subjective description of your own symptoms in order to make a decision about your need for a sleeping aid. It's up to you to be as open and honest as possible about your problem. If your sleep problem is more than a temporary side effect of a brief emotional upset or physical illness, you'll still have a sleep problem when you wake up after taking sleeping pills.

When used appropriately, however, prescription medications can be both effective and safe. Ideally, prescription sleep medications are limited to short-term use (7 to 10 days), after which you'll need to see your doctor again for a re-evaluation. There are several questions to ask your doctor if he or she prescribes a sleep medication for you:

➤ Why do you recommend this drug?

➤ How does the drug act to alleviate symptoms?

➤ What are the possible side effects?

➤ Will the drug interact with other medications I'm taking?

➤ What is the recommended schedule and dosage?

➤ Should I avoid alcohol while taking this medication?

➤ How long should I take it?

➤ What other steps can I take to solve my sleep problem?

By discussing the answers to these questions with your doctor, both of you can make an informed decision about which, if any, medication is right for your needs. You and your doctor should meet regularly to evaluate the effects and side effects of any medication you decide to take and to monitor the progress of your sleep problem.

Set Your Alarm!

Never stop taking prescription medication without first discussing the matter with your physician. You may need to taper off your use of the drug in order to prevent suffering serious side effects and withdrawal symptoms.

Although it's especially important to be aware of the actions and side effects of prescription medications, there are almost as many precautions to take when it comes to over-the-counter sleep aids (OTCs).

Over-the-Counter Herbs and Potions

The National Sleep Foundation estimates that about 40 percent of individuals suffering from insomnia self-medicate with OTCs or alcohol to hasten sleep. OTCs usually contain antihistamines that cause the same heavy-headed drowsiness that many cold medicines do. As discussed, antihistamines can also cause side effects, including dry mouth and dry eyes. If you take a large dose, or are particularly sensitive, sleepiness and even disorientation can last well into the next day.

It's important to be aware that side effects can creep up on you even with OTC medications. You may not realize how drowsy or disoriented you feel until you find yourself trying to cross the street against the light or attempting to sharpen a ball-point pen in the pencil sharpener. If you decide to take an OTC, pay special attention to how you feel the next day. If side effects are limited, and you experience only very occasional bouts of insomnia, then feel free to partake.

Set Your Alarm!

If you find yourself using a product more than once a week, talk to your doctor about the trouble you're having with sleep. Clearly, you'll need to address the underlying problem before you'll find a permanent solution.

Melatonin and tryptophan are two substances produced in the body that are known for their sleep-promoting properties. However, scientific literature offers a mixed assessment of melatonin's effectiveness and potential risks. And the history of tryptophan's use offers additional cautions.

Since neither melatonin nor tryptophan are legally considered drugs, they have not had to undergo the same kind of laboratory and clinical testing as substances considered medications. The Federal Drug Administration (FDA) does not have jurisdiction over naturally occurring substances, such as vitamins, amino acids, herbs, and hormones (like melatonin)—as long as their manufacturers make no health claims about them. If the manufacturers claim that melatonin is a "sleep aid," for instance, the FDA can consider it to be a drug and thus subject to the same strict rules and regulations used for prescription pharmaceuticals.

So far, however, melatonin, tryptophan, and most herbs (which we'll discuss later) remain outside the agency's purview. As a consumer, then, you need to conduct as much research about these products as you can by reading books like this one, talking to your doctor, and monitoring news reports about new studies conducted on these substances.

Melatonin: The "Dark" Hormone

Melatonin is a substance produced by the body's pineal gland, which lies at the base of the brain. Known as the "chemical expression of darkness," melatonin is produced almost exclusively at night, when it is dark. In healthy young adults, melatonin levels are lowest during the day, increase during the evening hours, and peak in the middle of the night.

As mentioned in Chapter 2, melatonin plays an important role in organizing daily circadian rhythms. High levels of the hormone send a biological signal to the brain to begin nighttime behavior, and decreasing levels signal the onset of daytime activity. As you get older, the amount of melatonin you produce diminishes, primarily because the pineal gland shrinks and calcifies with age. Some research indicates that one of the reasons older people have trouble staying asleep during the night is that they produce low levels of melatonin.

The theory behind using melatonin supplements—capsules, tablets, or liquids created in a laboratory—as a sleep aid is twofold: First, taking melatonin may help reset the body's clock by triggering the sleep response in the brain at a different time than it would normally occur. For this reason, many people find that taking melatonin helps them adjust to a new time zone more quickly than they would otherwise. Second, melatonin is also a sleep promoter; that is, a dose of melatonin before bedtime acts as a relatively immediate sleep aid in some people who take it—and, for most people, without any short-term side effects. (Since widespread use of melatonin supplements is relatively recent, a thorough exploration of its potential long-term side effects has not been completed.)

Rest Easy

Many melatonin supplements currently on the market come in tablets of up to 3 mg—over 10 times more than you need to reset your biological clock or to feel sleepy. We suggest that you buy brands that come in 1 mg doses and cut the tablet in half, and perhaps even into thirds, so that you take only 0.5 or 0.3 mg per night.

Unfortunately, researchers remain divided on what effects taking melatonin supplements really has on either disturbed biological rhythms or insomnia. There appears to be more evidence in favor of its use for jet lag and transient sleep/wake rhythm disorders.

It also remains unclear what, if any, dose of melatonin is best, when doses should be administered, and to whom. In fact, that's what makes it so tricky: Some people find that melatonin helps them fall asleep and stay asleep, while others experience no effect, and still others find it makes them feel groggy the next day—a hazardous side effect if there ever was one. Some people even report that melatonin causes them to feel too agitated and anxious to sleep.

Currently, melatonin supplements are available in various dosages—usually from 1 to 3 mg—in tablet or liquid form, which is more than your body produces in a day. Recent research suggests that you need far less than even the smallest dose to obtain results—only 0.3 mg, or a third of the 1 mg dose. Although melatonin supplements appear to be perfectly safe for most people in the short term, it's important to understand that melatonin is a powerful hormone, and even in small doses, it may affect a number of different body processes.

You should NOT take melatonin if you:

➤ Are pregnant, trying to get pregnant, or breast-feeding.

➤ Suffer from an autoimmune disease, diabetes, epilepsy, leukemia, or migraine headaches.

➤ Are taking cortisone medication.

➤ Are coping with kidney disease.

And, as we've said before, talk to your doctor before taking any sleeping aid.

Tryptophan

Studies of tryptophan's effects on sleep offer mixed results. According to Peter Hauri in his excellent book *No More Sleepless Nights* (Wiley, 1990), there are at least 25 studies suggesting that taking tryptophan supplements in the evening helps about half of all insomniacs—and that sometimes the supplements are even more effective than prescription medications. Other studies, however, show no such benefit.

To complicate matters, in 1988 and 1989 more than 1,500 people fell ill and 35 people died from a rare disorder called Eosinophilia Myalgia Syndrome, and their only common link was that they all used tryptophan to help them sleep. It appears that just one batch of tryptophan may have been contaminated during the manufacturing process and caused the syndrome to develop in those who took it. Nevertheless, this incident caused many doctors and patients alike to be wary of recommending and using tryptophan supplements.

If you want to see whether tryptophan will work for you, we recommend you try getting a dose of it from the foods you eat. As you may remember from Chapter 5, tryptophan is found in milk, meat, fish, eggs, and peanuts, so a glass of warm milk may do you as much good as taking a tryptophan supplement—and at far less risk.

The Herbal Route

In 1992, the U.S. National Institutes of Health, the federal government's largest supporter of medical research, announced the establishment of the Office of Alternative Medicine. Its goal remains to explore approaches to such chronic diseases as allergies, arthritis, heart disease—and, yes, insomnia—for which conventional Western medicine offers limited treatment options.

Among the most popular alternatives—and the one under a great deal of scrutiny by modern Western scientists—is the use of plants and plant material as medicine. Echinacea for colds, ginseng for anxiety and other conditions, and ginkgo biloba for Alzheimer's disease are just a few of the remedies that fall under the rubric of "herbal medicine."

Herbs as Medicine

Generally speaking, herbal medicines work in much the same way as do conventional pharmaceutical drugs. Herbs contain a large number of naturally occurring substances that work to alter the body's chemistry so it can return to its natural state of health. Unlike manufactured drugs, however, plants and other organic materials contain a wide variety of substances and, hence, less of any one particular active alkaloid. Herbs are thus less likely to be toxic to the body than are most pharmaceutical products.

Set Your Alarm!

Talk to an experienced herbalist before taking any herbs. Although herbs generally act gently on your body, they can cause side effects if taken in high doses or if you're particularly sensitive to them. Both hops and passionflower, for instance, can exacerbate depression in some people. Pay attention to how you react when you try a new remedy for any reason.

On the other hand, it's important to stress that herbs have only recently come under intense medical study, and thus we have few data on which to base either their effectiveness or their safety. Because the use of natural herbs has not come under the scrutiny of Western medicine for very long—and because many physicians have little experience using them with patients—definitive research about their benefits is relatively sparse. The good news is that, for most people, the risk of developing side effects from normal use is very small. Nevertheless, again, we want to stress caution when it comes to taking any substance— talk to your doctor before doing so.

Herbs for Insomnia

There are several herbs thought to help relax the body and induce sleep. Some are brewed to make teas, others are used as essential oils in the bath or dabbed on pillowcases. As discussed, however, the FDA does not regulate herbs— like vitamins, minerals, and other supplements, herbs are not treated as drugs. That means that you can't be absolutely sure of the strength, quality, or effectiveness of the products you buy. Seeking the help of a licensed practitioner of natural medicine or herbalist may help answer any questions you may have.

Before you read about the herbs useful for sleep, it's important to stress that in addition to any medicinal properties of the herbs themselves, you'll benefit from the ritual of preparation. Simply making a cup of warm tea or a warm bath part of your nightly ritual will aid you in your journey toward regular, restful sleep.

Among the most popular herbal remedies for insomnia are:

➤ **Chamomile** (Anthriscus cerefolium). Chamomile is used both as a tea and as a medicinal herb. You can buy chamomile tea in almost every grocery store, and you can buy chamomile flowers and leaves by mail order to make your own remedies. Some people claim that sleeping on a pillow stuffed with chamomile flowers, for example, makes for a particularly restful night's sleep.

➤ **Hops** (Humulus lupulus). Hops has been used as a
   flavoring and preservative in beer since the 9th century, and has had an even longer history as an
   herbal remedy for insomnia. The active ingredient
   in hops is lupulnic acid, which suppresses central
   nervous system activity and helps induce sleep.
   Hops is available in commercial herbal remedies as
   dried or fresh herbs from which to make a tea and in
   the form of capsules, powder, and tinctures. You can
   add drops of the tincture into boiling water and
   drink it like a tea.

➤ **Valerian** (Valerian officinalis). Quaintly known as
   the "Valium of the 19th century," valerian is widely
   recognized for its relaxing effect on the body. In
   Europe, doctors often prescribe it to treat anxiety. Its
   medicinal qualities are found in the root of the
   plant, which has a disagreeable odor. Fortunately,
   valerian is available as a pill or capsule, as well as a
   tincture. Most people prefer to take the pill because
   the roots have a bitter taste.

Prescription drugs, over-the-counter potions, and herbs
may help you to get some sorely needed sleep on an occasional basis, but if your sleep problem is chronic, you
need to know how to make it through a day when you
don't get your required amount of sleep the night before.
In the next chapter, we'll show you how.

Chapter 8

Staying Awake: Napping and Other Strategies

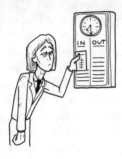

In This Chapter

➤ Exploring sleep deprivation and its effects

➤ The fine art of napping

➤ Tips for staying alert

According to a 1997 National Sleep Foundation/Gallup poll, more than 63 million Americans suffer dangerous levels of sleep deprivation, and nearly four in ten of those people reported that daytime sleepiness interferes with their day-to-day activities at least some of the time.

How about you? Did you take the Sleepiness Quotient Quiz in Chapter 1? How did you score? If you have any reason to believe that you're not getting enough sleep on a regular basis, and if you are attempting to function at optimal levels when your body is overtired, then read on. This chapter will help explain what happens when your body and brain go on the blink, and what you can do to prevent the worst from happening when they do. We'll also show you napping can help you prevent you from becoming sleep deprived. If you have trouble getting all the sleep you need at night, this chapter is written just for you.

Are You *Really* Alert?

Back in Chapter 5, we discussed the "fight-or-flight response," the physiological event that occurs when the body and mind senses danger. As you may remember, your sympathetic nervous system becomes activated in emergency situations, which causes your heart to beat faster, your blood pressure to rise, your muscles to tense up, and your respiration rate to increase. When these physiological responses occur, your body is at its most alert and active: You're literally wide awake and ready for anything. But you have another part of your nervous system that takes over when the emergency has been resolved. The *parasympathetic nervous system* causes you to relax: It slows down your heart and respiration rates, lowers your blood pressure, and relaxes your muscles. And the more relaxed you are, the less alert you are.

Words to Sleep By

The **parasympathetic nervous system** is the part of the autonomic nervous system responsible for relaxing or slowing down the body's activities after they have been stimulated by the sympathetic nervous system.

When it comes to making it through a day (or night) when you're feeling sleepy, you'll want to do your best to "switch on" the sympathetic nervous system and "switch off" its counterpart, the parasympathetic nervous system. We'll show you how to do that later in the chapter.

Measuring Alertness

How do you know when you're alert, when you're drowsy, or when you're about to fall asleep? And how do you know when your level of alertness is about to dip below the safety level? You might find those questions pretty hard to answer, and if so, you're not alone. Even laboratory tests designed to measure and evaluate alertness have trouble isolating the elements involved in these conditions. The standard laboratory test used to assess alertness today is the Multiple Sleep Latency Test (MSLT),which determines the time it takes a person to fall asleep in a darkened room. A person with a very low alertness level will drop off in less than five minutes or so, while an alert person will spend the entire allotted bed time of 20 minutes wide awake.

When combined with information about how much the subject slept the night before, the MSLT allows us to put numbers on the relative effects of the loss of sleep. The following figures show what happens to alertness if you lose just two hours of sleep each night.

Indeed, the loss of just a few hours of sleep can considerably reduce your level of alertness just when you may need it most. You've read some of the statistics about the high costs of sleep deprivation in Chapter 1, but it's important to reiterate some of them here. Did you know, for instance, that the primary cause of the Three Mile Island accident, in which a Pennsylvania nuclear power plant nearly experienced a core meltdown, was operator carelessness and inattention in the wee hours of the morning?

Without question, fatigued people make errors. And while most of these errors are on a much smaller scale than the

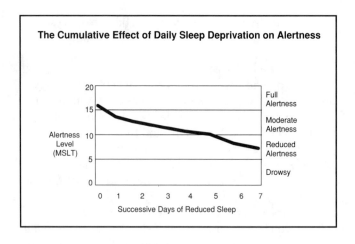

The Cumulative Effect of Daily Sleep Deprivation on Alertness

This graph shows the cumulative effects of a loss of just two hours of sleep every night over the course of a week. The first day after such a loss you might not fare so poorly, but by the fifth, sixth, or seventh day, your alertness level has fallen to a dangerous level.

Three Mile Island disaster, taken together they have an enormous effect. Remember, when the body and brain fail to get the rest they need, certain functions become impaired. You can't concentrate as well, your reaction time is slower, your creative juices certainly aren't flowing, and your mood, well, that's just shot. Sometimes you merely get through your day on "automatic pilot." You simply go through the motions without really thinking about them. Unfortunately, this phenomenon, known as *automatic behavior,* is probably the real reason that so many accidents occur to sleep-deprived people. Examples of automatic behavior include a railroad engineer who can continue pressing a safety lever at regular intervals but doesn't notice an obstruction on the track, and a trucker who keeps his rig on the road but misses his intended exit.

Words to Sleep By

Automatic behavior refers to a period of several seconds to minutes when a sleep-deprived person is able to continue performing routine duties but is incapable of active cognition—which means he or she can carry out a task without thinking about what's really occurring at the time.

The Drive to Sleep

Drowsy driving is all sleep too common, especially among young men aged 25 and under. Night-shift workers who rotate their schedules are also at high risk, a fact we'll discuss in more depth in Chapter 12. Others at risk include people who regularly drive long distances, such as truck drivers, and those who have insomnia or other sleep problems.

Here are some of the symptoms of drowsy driving:

➤ Your eyes go out of focus or close.

➤ You have trouble keeping your head up.

➤ You can't stop yawning.

➤ You have trouble concentrating.

➤ You realize you don't remember driving the last few miles.

➤ You drift between lanes, tailgate, or miss traffic signs.

➤ You drift off the road or narrowly miss crashing.

A little later in this chapter you'll learn some general tips about staying awake during the day. In the meantime, here are some tips specifically designed to help you drive safely at any hour:

➤ **Rest up.** Get enough sleep the night before, and plan to drive during times of the day when you normally feel most alert and awake.

➤ **Choose your time wisely.** Avoid driving during your body's "down times," which are, for Regular Robins, during the mid-afternoon and then between midnight and 6 a.m.

➤ **Drive with a buddy.** Not only can you share driving responsibilities, but you can also monitor each other's signs of drowsiness and help each other stay awake. When driving through the night, BOTH of you should stay awake. If your buddy goes to sleep while you're driving, there's no one left to monitor your level of alertness.

➤ **Take breaks.** Schedule a break every two hours or every 100 miles—but stop sooner if you show any danger signs of sleepiness. During your break, stretch, take a walk, and eat a light snack before getting back into the car. If you're sleepy, take a 10- or 20-minute nap.

Set Your Alarm!

For safety's sake, if you need to stop driving to catch a nap, do so only in a safe, well-lit, heavily-trafficked travel plaza or truck stop—and always lock your doors.

Read on for more tips, some of which you can use to help you stay alert while driving.

The Fine Art of Napping

Cats and babies: For many people, these are the only creatures who do (or should) nap on a regular basis. But nothing could be further from the truth. Built into the human circadian hardware are two major opportunities for sleep: one in the middle of the night and the other in mid-afternoon. For many people, taking a nap either on a regular basis or in order to make up for a sleep debt helps them function well throughout the day and, indeed, sleep better at night.

What about you? What did you find out about your napping nature back in Chapter 3? Can you—and do you—easily nap to make up for a sleep loss or to prepare for a particularly long night or day ahead? Or do you think napping is simply not part of your nature? (If you're really nap-o-phobic, you probably think napping is a waste of time no matter who's doing the napping!)

The fact is, if you really aren't getting the sleep that you need at night, you probably *can* learn to nap efficiently. In this chapter, we'll explore the nature of napping and then show you how to build a nap into your day.

Who Naps?

The practice ofsleep deprivation napping has developed in many cultures around the world. You've no doubt heard of the "siesta"—the lovely Mediterranean and Latin American tradition of taking a post-lunch afternoon nap. In Mexico, for example, about 80 percent of adults indulge in an almost daily 90-minute nap. The siesta may have developed, at least in part, to give workers a rest during the hottest part of the afternoon, as well as to provide them with enough energy to work later into the evening hours.

According to the 1997 National Sleep Foundation/Gallup Poll "Sleepiness in America," only about one in five Americans report that they take regular naps. Indeed, there remains a resistance to napping in our culture, even though sleep deprivation has become a major problem throughout the nation. In fact, although planned napping is apparently anathema to American go-getters, unplanned napping—while driving, while working, while at school—seems to be on the rise, leading to the loss of life as well as millions of dollars in lost productivity.

Fortunately, more and more companies are beginning to see the advantages of allowing—even encouraging—planned napping in the workplace. Especially helpful for night-shift and split-shift workers in 24-hour companies, napping as a strategy for increasing productivity is also showing up in industries that demand a high level of creativity, including advertising agencies, software development companies, and investment houses. Because judicious napping refreshes the creative mind and helps relieve stress, workers who "indulge" at the right time can then put in longer hours before losing motivation and inspiration.

Nevertheless, we've got a long way to go before most Americans consider napping a worthy enterprise and a habit worth cultivating. The signs are good, however, that the tide is turning. Napping rooms devoid of phones, faxes, or computer screens and equipped with cots or napping chairs are popping up in more and more workplaces every day.

The Truth About Napping

Our resistance to napping here in the United States appears to be as much a part of our own culture as the siesta is in other societies. In fact, our "work through anything" mentality has spawned a few myths about napping that deserve to be dispelled here and now. These myths include:

➤ **To want to nap is an inherent sign of laziness.** First of all, you already know that you have a built-in, physiological desire for a nap in the mid-afternoon. While some people hardly feel that urge, or can suppress it quite easily, those of us who accept it (even relish it) are no less healthy or motivated.

➤ **If you nap during the day, you won't sleep well at night.** This is one of the oldest myths about napping around. The truth is, napping during the day— if you're sleep-deprived—can actually help you sleep *better* at night! Consider this: After having had a poor night's sleep and a long, busy day, have you ever then simply felt too anxious and stressed to sleep when you finally get to bed at night? That feeling can make it impossible for you to fall asleep and stay asleep. If you'd had a nap earlier that day, on the other hand, your body and mind would be under less stress and far more able to relax and sleep at night.

➤ **Mid-afternoon is the only time you're supposed to nap.** While the mid-afternoon (around 2 or 3 p.m.) is when most people find it easiest to nap, no specific time is completely off-limits. Remember, we each have our own unique internal clocks that help to set our daily rhythms. Remember Oliver the Owl, whom you met in Chapter 3? The times he would prefer to nap are very different from his Lark counterpart, Letitia. And a Regular Robin may have a much more flexible napping ability than his Owl and Lark counterparts. If you listen to your own body and take advantage of its natural lulls and dips, you'll be able to find the most comfortable and successful time to nap for you. Avoid napping within a few hours of your bedtime, however, which can keep you up at night.

➤ **Long naps are better than short naps.** Although it may seem unlikely, the truth is that a 15- to 30-minute nap can be just as refreshing in certain situations as a longer nap of 90 to 100 minutes—and it will clearly be superior to one that lasts from 45 minutes to an hour. That's because of the architecture of sleep (described in Chapter 2)—at 45 minutes, you are half-way through the 90-minute sleep cycle and in the deepest stages of sleep. Indeed, carefully timing a nap to make it either very short or long can make all the difference in the world.

Timing Your Naps

Drowsiness, then deeper and deeper sleep, then a state of active but unconscious brain activity, then almost awake again, and then back down into deep sleep—so goes the sleep cycle, which takes about 90 to 100 minutes. We travel through this remarkable cycle several times a night.

What you might not realize is that the 90-minute sleep cycle is part of a larger pattern of rest and activity that continues throughout the day. Known as the basic rest-activity cycle, or BRAC, this pattern explains why there are times when you feel especially alert and times when you're desperate for a cup of caffeine or a burst of fresh air to stimulate you. These "down times" represent the times when the circuits complete more slowly, when the vestiges of a catnapping ancestry show through. The BRAC cycles are usually very subtle, and we are usually able to either ignore them or to compensate for them with caffeine or other forms of stimulation. (It's no accident that the typical workplace coffee break takes place at 10:30, 90 minutes after work begins and, for many people, 180 minutes after getting out of bed at 7:30.)

Although the BRAC pattern is most pronounced at night when you'd normally be in bed asleep, you also experience it during the day. Becoming aware of your daily fluctuations up and down the alertness wave (see the following figure) will help you find the best naptime for your body and mind. In fact, there are two reasons to understand the 90-minute rhythm: First, you'll be able to better choose a time when you're more likely to fall asleep. Second, you'll know about how long to sleep in order to wake up feeling refreshed and ready to go instead of groggy and out-of-sorts.

The best time to start to nap during any 90-minute cycle is at the point when you first start to feel drowsy. . .not when you're already having trouble keeping your eyes open. If you get into napping position and close your eyes at that time, your body and mind can take full advantage of the 10- or 20-minute down-swing of alertness during that cycle. If you can afford it and are particularly sleep-deprived, you could sleep for a whole 90 minutes, going through all four stages of sleep plus a whole REM (dreaming cycle).

However—and this is a big however—if you can't make it through a whole sleep cycle, you'll want to limit your nap to just 10 to 30 minutes. That way, you won't interrupt the deepest stages of non-REM sleep, which can leave you feeling worse than when you started. In fact, there's a strange thing that happens when you're awakened from a deep sleep called *sleep inertia*. Your arms and legs feel paralyzed, your vision is blurry, and you have difficulty concentrating. Sleep inertia usually lasts only about 30 minutes or so, but some people who wake up like this feel off-kilter for the rest of the day. Timing your sleep period so that you don't wake up during a non-REM cycle is the best way to avoid sleep inertia.

Words to Sleep By

Sleep inertia is the term used to describe a set of symptoms usually related to waking up from the deep stages of sleep.

Although it may seem complicated at first, with a little practice you can learn to nap when your body and mind most crave a break, and then wake up feeling refreshed and ready to go. By timing your naps this way you'll help yourself avoid the dangers and the discomfort of sleep inertia.

Defining Your Napping Style

Winston Churchill went all the way, stripping down to his skivvies and climbing into bed for a nap that lasted a good hour and a half. Other nappers simply lean back in their chairs, close their eyes, and drift off to sleep for just 10 or 15 minutes.

How, when, and, indeed, if you nap depends on your Nap-Ability, as well as other aspects of your Sleep Personality, as assessed in Chapter 3. Take another look at how you scored, then read on to find out how best to incorporate naps into your life.

Generally speaking, the best time to doze is mid-afternoon. That's when our alertness levels are normally at their lowest and, if we're running a little short of sleep, it's easiest and most refreshing to nap at that time. But that's just a general rule because each of us has a special Sleep Personality that helps determine if, when, and how we nap:

➤ **Long Sleepers.** Obtaining nine or ten uninterrupted hours of sleep—what long sleepers crave and require—is often impossible, especially for working parents or people who want to have an evening social life but who have to get up early in the morning for work. For long sleepers short on available night time, an afternoon or early-evening nap can make up the difference and keep them feeling alert and refreshed.

Set Your Alarm!

Monitor the effects of naps on your nighttime sleep with care. If you find it hard to sleep at night but nap nearly every day, you may want to cut down on, or cut out, your daytime naps. Remember, you only need to sleep a certain number of hours each day to feel rested and alert. Too long a nap at the wrong time (especially within a few hours of bedtime) is bound to affect the quality of your major sleep period at night.

➤ **Short Sleepers.** Those of you who consistently get less than six hours of sleep per night could probably use the boost you get from grabbing a bit of shut-eye at some point during the day—and you probably could use that boost on a regular basis. However, if you feel awake and alert throughout the day, you shouldn't feel *obligated* to nap just because you naturally sleep less than the "norm" of seven hours. Again, let your natural rhythms and needs help you determine a sleep/wake, rest/activity schedule that works for you.

➤ **Split Sleepers.** There are people out there who quite naturally (or at least easily) divide their wake periods into two portions, pretty much on a daily basis. They may sleep four to six hours during the night, then, about eight hours later, sleep another one to three hours. In essence, split sleepers live two "mini" days in the course of a single regular one and enjoy a restful, rejuvenating sleep period in-between each of their eight-hour days. As you can imagine, split sleepers are perfect night workers, and can easily adapt to time-zone changes.

➤ **Rigid Larks.** Remember Letitia the Lark, who simply couldn't sleep later in the morning no matter what time she got to bed at night? For Rigid Larks like her, taking a nap to either make up for a loss of sleep or prepare the body for a later-than-usual night is an essential strategy to avoid sleep deprivation.

➤ **Night Owls.** Oliver the Owl and his late-night brethren, on the other hand, make up for losses they suffer when having to get up earlier than usual by taking short naps in the evening. Oliver takes a 20-minute nap around 8 p.m., which refreshes him enough to make it through to his usual bedtime of about midnight. If he goes to bed for the night when he's exhausted at 8 or 9 p.m., on the other hand, he's liable to sleep until 1 a.m. and then be up all night.

➤ **Regular Robins.** Some Regular Robins (those people who have relatively "normal" sleep schedules that start between about 11 p.m. and midnight and finish at 6:30 or 7:30 a.m.) stay "regular" by taking a nap whenever they feel sleep-deprived. They aren't split sleepers, however, so naps are rarely a regular part of their routine. In most cases, Regular Robins are best able to nap in the mid-afternoon.

Tips for Healthy Napping

No matter who you are or when you nap, it's just as important to practice good sleep hygiene during these shorter sleep periods as it is at night. Here are some tips to help you become a better napper:

➤ **Stick to a routine.** As much as possible, get your body "in the mood" for a nap by following a pre-nap routine. If it's a short nap you're aiming for, performing a few simple stretches and loosening your tie or collar might be enough. If you're going for a long nap, you might want to follow (as much as possible) the same pre-bed routine you do at night—brushing your teeth, reading for a few minutes, and so on. This routine can even work at the office, as long as it doesn't involve changing into your pj's and clutching your teddy bear.

➤ **Batten down the hatches.** Even if you're taking a short 10- or 20-minute nap, take a few minutes (starting as soon as you feel drowsy) to turn off the lights, unplug the phone, and get as comfortable as possible. If you're taking a 90-minute nap, it's especially important to free your environment of all distractions.

➤ **Take advantage of your napping "windows of opportunity."** Once you start to feel drowsy, you're on the down-swing of a BRAC (basic rest-activity cycle). At that point, your body is ready to nap. If you try to nap when you're feeling alert, on the other hand, chances are you simply won't be able to, no matter how sleep-deprived you are.

➤ **Go short or long.** Again, you want to avoid that middle ground—the 40- or 50-minute nap that interrupts your deepest stages of sleep or your REM cycle. Otherwise you risk waking up feeling groggy and out-of-sorts—just the symptoms you wanted to avoid by taking a nap. Unless you can go for the whole 90 minutes, set an alarm clock to wake you after 10 or 20 minutes.

And there you have it: napping strategies for every Sleep Personality—and that includes yours. As you head into the 21st century along with the rest of us, it's likely the demands on your time will become even greater and more pressing. It's essential—for your health and sanity—to keep your body and mind as rested and refreshed as possible. Indeed, napping may be the "wonder drug" of the new millennium!

Rest Easy

If you know you're going to have a very late night—or even pull an all-nighter for one reason or another—you can take a "prophylactic" nap during the afternoon. Studies show that taking a 90-minute nap before staying awake all night increases alertness and performance by about 30 percent.

In the best of all possible worlds, you'd get all the sleep you need every night, work regular hours throughout your career, never have to care for an infant or parent in the middle of the night, and thus wake up every day feeling terrific.

But you're in the real world, aren't you? And so you have days when you're just not feeling your best after a night of restless sleep, days that nonetheless require you to be every bit as perky and efficient as you would be with a full night's sleep. On days like that, you need some help, don't you? Well, that's what we're here for. Here are some tips we hope will help you make the most of those kinds of days:

➤ **Rise to the challenge.** Performing a boring, routine task when you're already feeling drowsy just about puts you over the edge, doesn't it? But if you've got something new and preferably stimulating to do, you're apt to perk right up. In Chapter 12, we'll talk about how urgent such stimulation is when it comes to safety-sensitive jobs, such as those in the nuclear power industry. In the meantime, if you find yourself losing focus, switch to a more refreshing task until you feel better.

➤ **Move it or lose it.** Any type of muscular activity triggers the sympathetic nervous system and helps keep you alert—and you don't have to run a mile or lift weights for the activity to have a positive effect. Depending on how sleep-deprived you are, walking around the block or performing simple stretches at your desk may be enough to boost your alertness level for an hour or two. Even chewing gum can briefly give you a lift.

➤ **Cool off.** A blast of cool dry air helps raise your alertness level, especially if you've been lulled into drowsiness by sitting in a warm, humid environment. Open a window, run a fan, or—if you have this option—take a cool shower.

➤ **Aromatherapy 101.** Some researchers believe that aroma can play a role in enhancing alertness. For instance, a driving simulation study by the Institute for Circadian Physiology published in *Sleep Research* found that the scent of peppermint "had an alerting effect at the end of the night when the subjects were most sleepy." In this study, six volunteers drove during the overnight hours on two different nights. On one night, a peppermint scent was diffused into the driving simulation room every ten minutes for two seconds. The drivers were exposed to unscented air the second night. The volunteers scored better on the night that they were exposed to the scent of peppermint.

➤ **Always eat breakfast.** If you don't eat breakfast, your body will be operating at an energy deficit when you need the fuel most.

➤ **Combine complex carbohydrates and protein.** A low-sugar, high-fiber cereal and low-fat milk or yogurt is a perfect meal for those just getting ready to go—the combination makes for long-lasting energy.

➤ **Avoid the high-sugar/high-carbohydrate rush.** Consuming sugar and carbohydrates like those found in doughnuts or pastries will trigger an energy rush at first, but then you'll crash. Carbohydrates, especially in combination with fat, trigger the release of serotonin, which will help calm you, but may also make you sleepy.

➤ **Monitor caffeine intake.** Although the first thing you reach for is a cup of coffee or tea when you're feeling sleepy, consuming too much caffeine can cause wild rises and dips in energy and mood, especially if you do so continuously on a daily basis. Limit your intake to one or two cups in the morning and one or two during your afternoon slump if you feel the need.

Staying Awake and Alert

We hope this chapter has given you some tips about staying awake and alert throughout the day, no matter how little sleep you obtained the night before. Clearly, however, it's better to get the sleep you need during the night (or the day if you work at night). For those of you who snore—or sleep with someone who does—that's easier said than done. That's what we'll discuss next in Chapter 9.

To Sleep, Perchance to Snore

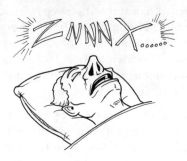

In This Chapter

➤ Understanding snoring and sleep apnea

➤ Defining the risks and side effects of sleep apnea

➤ Exploring some solutions to snoring and sleep apnea

"Laugh and the world laughs with you. Snore, and you sleep alone." So goes perhaps the most famous and eloquent observation, made by author Anthony Burgess, about this very common—and very disruptive—sleep problem. A potent destroyer of the marriage bed and the subject of endless jokes and comedy bits, snoring can be either a mild annoyance or a sign of a serious health condition. In fact, snoring and its close relative, Obstructive Sleep Apnea, represent the most common sleep problems in the United States.

In this chapter, we'll help all you snorers—and your partners—gain some insight into your problem, determine its severity, and offer some potential solutions.

The Big Snore

Ranging from the gentle rumble of an undercurrent to a raging, snorting cacophony, the sounds of snoring disturb millions of households every night. (And snoring can be dangerous to your health in more ways than one: Legend has it that infamous Texas gunfighter John Wesley Hardin killed a snorer who disturbed his sleep by shooting him through the wall of his adjoining hotel room.) Today, snoring is extremely common. About 25 percent of all men snore each night, while about half as many women snore. Unusual among young people, the prevalence of snoring increases after the age of 35.

Plainly speaking, snoring is a noise produced when an individual breathes during sleep (usually when the sleeper breathes *in*). This sound occurs as air is forced through the narrow air passage. This forced passage of air, in turn, causes the soft palate and uvula (you know, that thing that hangs down in the back of your throat) to vibrate. Sometimes, vibrations of the tongue, tonsils, and sides of the throat also contribute to the sound of snoring.

In addition to so-called "simple snoring," there is a medical condition—a potentially quite serious one—called Obstructive Sleep Apnea. With sleep apnea, a sleep disorder suffered by about 2 to 4 percent of middle-aged adults, the upper airway becomes completely obstructed for 10 seconds or longer, and often many times—sometimes hundreds of times—during the night. Although it's a serious medical disorder, more than 80 percent of sleep apneics fail to understand the problem or get medical help for it. And that's unfortunate because successful treatment can mean significant relief.

The relationship between snoring and sleep apnea is a close one. By definition, all sleep apneics snore. Furthermore, recent research suggests that, over time, simple snoring can damage the tissues in the throat and nasal passages, making the development of sleep apnea more likely. As we'll discuss in this chapter, both snoring and sleep apnea can have serious health consequences and should never be taken lightly.

The Physiology of Snoring

Although most bed partners believe that snoring is simply a dastardly plot to keep them awake in the most annoying way possible, people who snore are anatomically different than their non-snoring counterparts. Among the differences that help create the problem—differences that are more pronounced in those with Obstructive Sleep Apnea than in simple snorers—are:

> ➤ **Poor muscle tone in the muscles of the tongue and throat.** This condition allows the tongue to fall backwards into the airway or the sides of the throat to close together.

> ➤ **Excessive bulkiness of the throat.** Being overweight and having a large neck size often contribute to snoring. Large tonsils and adenoids also commonly cause snoring in children.

> ➤ **Excessive length of the soft palate and uvula.** A long palate may narrow the opening from the nose into the throat. As it dangles in the airway, it acts as a flutter valve during relaxed breathing and contributes to the noise of snoring. A long uvula may make matters even worse.

> ➤ **Obstructed nasal airways.** When you have a stuffy or blocked-up nose, you have to inhale even harder to get enough air into your lungs. This creates an exaggerated vacuum in the throat—the collapsible part of the airway—that pulls together the floppy tissues of the throat. This phenomenon explains why some people snore only during hay fever season or when they have a cold or sinus infection.

In most cases, snoring is fairly simple and straightforward. It isn't horribly loud or raucous and it doesn't wake you up or disturb your sleep. Now, that doesn't mean that even simple snoring can't be serious: If it bothers your bed partner, it's serious. You may slumber the night away and wake up feeling refreshed, while your bedmate tosses and turns for hours and suffers from sleep deprivation the next day.

Rest Easy

If your partner's snoring keeps you awake at night, you MUST take action in order to avoid chronic sleep deprivation yourself. In addition to showing him or her this chapter, you can buy earplugs or sleep in another room until your partner finds a solution to the snoring problem.

Diagnosing Sleep Apnea

This quiz will help you decide if your snoring is a mere annoyance or a potential health hazard. Again, please note that some recent research suggests that simple snoring may eventually lead to sleep apnea in some people.

Is It Snoring or Sleep Apnea?

1. Does your snoring disturb your bed partner?

   Never ____ Sometimes ____ Usually ____

2. Do you snore in all sleeping positions?

   Never ____ Sometimes ____ Usually ____

3. Do you ever wake suddenly because of snoring?

   Never ____ Sometimes ____ Usually ____

4. Are you tired when you have to get up in the morning?

   Never ____ Sometimes ____ Usually ____

5. Are you tired during the day?

   Never ____ Sometimes ____ Usually ____

6. Do you fall asleep while at the movies, watching TV, or while listening to a lecture?

   Never ____ Sometimes ____ Usually ____

7. Do you stop breathing for several seconds between snores (you'll probably have to ask a bed partner for the answer to this question!)?

   Never ____ Sometimes ____ Usually ____

Score yourself 1 point for every "Never," 2 points for every "Sometimes," and 3 points for every "Usually." If you scored between 7 and 10 points, your snoring falls into the mild annoyance category. If you scored between 11 and 15, your snoring is probably disturbing you and your bed partner and may require treatment. A score between 16 and 21 means that your snoring is significantly disrupting your sleep and may be putting you at risk for more serious problems.

The Truth About Sleep Apnea

Sleep apnea is more than just loud snoring. If you suffer from this medical condition, you literally stop breathing while asleep. In most cases, a condition called *Obstructive Sleep Apnea* is the problem. What happens is that your tongue or other soft tissues fall back and either completely collapse or partially obstruct the airway. Oxygen levels drop, and your throat muscles contract as you struggle to breathe. This break can last from a few seconds up to a minute or even longer. Finally, your throat opens, and you gasp or let out a snort as air rushes in. You then fall back asleep.

Words to Sleep By

Obstructive Sleep Apnea is a condition in which breathing temporarily stops during sleep because the tongue and other tissues block the back of the throat.

Those with severe cases of sleep apnea repeat this process dozens of times each hour, up to 500 or more times a night. If you suffer from sleep apnea, snorting and snoring may become such a part of the nightly routine that you have no memory of your spasmodic breathing or its effect on your sleep.

In addition to Obstructive Sleep Apnea, two other forms of the condition exist:

➤ **Central Sleep Apnea.** This fairly rare condition affects mostly adults over the age of 60. The brain "forgets" to tell the breathing muscles to move, and thus the sleeper stops breathing for several seconds until he or she wakes up and starts breathing again.

➤ **Mixed Sleep Apnea.** This condition involves brief periods of Central Sleep Apnea followed by longer periods of Obstructive Sleep Apnea.

Sleep Apnea: The Symptoms

Again, sleep apnea is more than just loud or constant snoring. It is related to a host of often serious medical conditions. The risks associated with sleep apnea include:

➤ **Excessive daytime sleepiness.** Because their breathing problems cause them to wake up several times a night, sleep apneics suffer terribly from sleep deprivation. In addition to physical, social, and psychological discomfort, such sleepiness can result in serious traffic and on-the-job accidents.

➤ **Irregular heartbeat.** With each episode of apnea, the heart rate falls, then increases again at the termination of apnea. In a small number of cases (about 3 percent), a serious arrhythmia (irregular heart rhythm) develops.

➤ **High blood pressure.** Several studies show an increased risk of high blood pressure in people with sleep apnea, and they are more frequently diagnosed with high blood pressure than their healthy counterparts.

➤ **Heart disease and stroke.** Sleep apnea has been associated with an increased incidence of heart attacks and stroke. Sleep lab evaluations of male stroke patients show that 75 percent of them have significantly increased numbers of apneic events.

The relationship between cardiovascular disease (including high blood pressure, heart disease, and stroke) and sleep apnea is currently under investigation by the National Heart, Lung, and Blood Institute. The Institute is conducting a Sleep Heart Health Study in which the sleep patterns and habits of 6,000 Americans, 40 years and older, will be examined to see what, if any, connection exists between sleep apnea and cardiovascular disease. The study, which began in 1995, will be completed later this year.

Despite these severe related conditions, the symptoms of sleep apnea may be vague and subtle. You may feel tired and sleepy during the day, even after what you perceive to be a full night's sleep. You may have a headache, feel irritable, and experience memory difficulties and problems with concentration. Depression, impotence or loss of sex drive, and anxiety are also common side effects.

Are You at Risk?

Obstructive Sleep Apnea is most common in middle age and more likely to strike men than women. One big risk factor appears to be body fat. Sixty percent of people with sleep apnea are overweight. Specifically, however, it is not the excess poundage, but the neck size that counts. Men with a neck circumference of 17 inches or larger—16 inches for women—are more likely to have their airways collapse while they sleep. So are people with double chins or with a lot of fat at the waist. Apnea usually worsens with age because the tissues in the throat become floppier, and people tend to gain weight at this time. Men are more susceptible because they often have beefier throat tissues and are more likely to gather fat in their abdomen, neck, and shoulders than women—all factors that contribute to creating a narrower airway.

Set Your Alarm!

You may not be aware that you suffer from Obstructive Sleep Apnea. The condition may cause only mild disturbances in your sleep—disrupting your normal cycle but not causing you to wake up and open your eyes. In fact, you may be completely unaware that you even have a problem.

There may be a genetic link as well. Snoring does run in families, and relatives of those affected with apnea tend to be more likely to have apnea and shallow breathing.

Solving Sleep Apnea

If you think you may suffer from sleep apnea, talk to your doctor. He or she may suggest that you spend a night in a sleep laboratory to undergo special testing. Along with monitoring the stages of sleep you pass through and how long they last, the lab staff will measure your blood oxygen saturation, or the amount of oxygen your blood is carrying through your body, which indicates how much oxygen you inhale during sleep. They'll measure your respiration and also use an *oximeter,* which transmits a beam of light through a finger, toe, or ear and measures the wavelength of light that passes through. This measurement indicates the percentage of oxygen in the blood. Generally speaking, the less oxygen in the blood, the more severe your sleep apnea is likely to be: It means that you're not breathing in enough oxygen while you sleep.

Words to Sleep By

An **oximeter** is a device used to measure blood oxygen levels, an important diagnostic indicator of sleep apnea. The less oxygen in your blood, the more severely apnea is affecting your ability to breathe.

Once you know that you have sleep apnea and doctors have determined its severity, you can decide on the most appropriate treatment. Currently, the most effective treatment for moderate to severe sleep apnea is the CPAP, or Continuous Positive Airway Pressure. This device works during sleep by blowing air from a machine into a mask that you place over your nose. The air pressure keeps your airway open, thus eliminating the apnea and frequent awakenings. Once you can breathe normally during the night, you'll start to feel better almost immediately. Indeed, symptoms of daytime alertness often significantly improve after just one night and are completely back to normal in a week or two. Unfortunately, you have to continue to use CPAP throughout your life, unless you can lose sufficient weight or are one of the limited number of people who benefit from surgery.

These remarkable results tend to make up for the major drawback of CPAP, namely the mild discomfort the device causes at first. Most people get used to this setup quickly, however, especially when they realize how much better they feel during the day.

In some cases, your doctor may recommend surgery to treat your severe snoring and apnea. One technique, called the *uvuloplatopharyngoplasy,* or UPPP, reduces the size of the uvula, soft palate, or both. Only 50 percent of apneics have success with this technique. It is expensive and involves a painful recovery period. Another surgical procedure zaps away excess tissue with a laser. Called a laser-assisted *uvulopalatoplasty,* or LAUP, this procedure is less costly and requires a shorter and less painful recovery period than UPPP. On the downside, it often requires several treatments before it's effective. An even newer procedure, somnoplasty, achieves the same end result (less excess tissue and reduced size of uvula) using microwaves.

Words to Sleep By

A **uvuloplatopharyngoplasy** is a surgical procedure that's used to reduce the size of the uvula, soft palate, or both. A **uvulopalatoplasty** is a laser surgery technique used to remove excess tissue from the back of the throat to reduce snoring and apnea.

Finding the Answer to Snoring

Snoring is not the easiest condition to cure, as the sheer
number of devices and techniques developed to do so indicate. Indeed, more than 300 devices are registered in the
U.S. Patent and Trademark Office as cures for snoring.
Some are variations on the old idea of sewing a tennis ball
on the pajama back to force the sleeper to avoid a back
sleeping position, which tends to exacerbate snoring (see
the following tip). Chin and head straps, neck collars, and
devices inserted into the mouth are other options, though
these may prove ineffective for your particular case. Many
electrical devices have been designed to produce painful
or unpleasant stimuli when snoring occurs. Again, the
success rate is not remarkable, but some people do find
that one or more of these gadgets can help.

Here are some healthful options for you to try (such as
losing weight and cutting down on alcohol) and others
that may or may not help your particular situation:

> ➤ **Lose weight if you need to.** Even a relatively small
>   loss in weight—say, 10 to 15 pounds—can make a
>   difference when it comes to snoring and Obstructive
>   Sleep Apnea.

> ➤ **Change position.** Most snorers tend to sleep on
>   their backs. If you do, try sleeping on your side or
>   stomach to see if that makes a difference.

> ➤ **Avoid alcohol and tranquilizers.** These substances
>   relax throat muscle tissue and depress breathing,
>   thus making both snoring and apnea more likely.

> ➤ **Stop smoking.** Cigarette smoke can swell throat tis-
>   sues, increase mucus formation, and worsen the low
>   oxygen levels that accompany apnea.

> ➤ **Clear up stuffiness.** If you have a cold or suffer from
>   allergies, use a decongestant that helps clear your
>   nasal passages and makes it easier for you to breathe.

➤ **Use a dental appliance.** A dentist can fit you with an oral device that repositions your tongue and jaw to hold them forward. Because it keeps the tongue from closing against the back of the throat, you may find such a device helpful. According to the August 1995 issue of *Sleep,* such devices help about 60 percent of people who have Obstructive Sleep Apnea.

➤ **Try a "snore alarm."** At least one company (Sharper Image) sells a wrist-watch that monitors snoring and wakes you up with a silent alarm of powerful vibrations that begin as soon as you start to snore.

No matter what, it's important that you don't give up when it comes to finding a solution to your snoring problem. If you consistently snore and suffer from sleep deprivation, get yourself to a doctor for an evaluation. If you're diagnosed with sleep apnea, persevere until you find a treatment that works for you. Not only will your bed partner thank you for giving him or her the chance for consistent good sleep, but you'll be improving your health as well as your daytime alertness levels.

Rest Easy

To avoid rolling over on your back during the night, try stuffing a tennis ball into a sock and clip it to the back of your nightshirt.

We hope these suggestions help you—and your partner— get a better night's sleep. In the next chapter, we'll discuss another set of sleep disorders—including sleepwalking and talking, teeth grinding, and two related syndromes called Restless Leg Movement Disorder and Periodic Leg Movement Disorder—that also disrupt sleep.

Chapter 10

Sleep Disorders 101

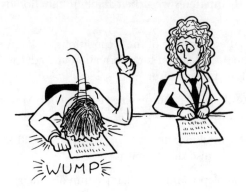

≋WUMP≋

In This Chapter

➤ Restless Leg Syndrome and Periodic Limb Movement Disorder

➤ The sleep "paranormals": night terrors, sleep-walking, sleeptalking, and REM behavior disorder

➤ The signs and symptoms of narcolepsy

➤ Understanding circadian rhythms disorders

➤ Ways to enjoy quiet, still nights of sleep—at the right time

A swift kick to the calf, the sound of grinding teeth, the thought that a child might wander out of bed into a dangerous situation—these and other nighttime events disturb the sleep of countless people throughout the world. Millions of other people suffer from another type of sleep disorder: They take their sleep at the wrong time because the "hardwiring" of their internal clocks has somehow gone haywire. They may experience such severe daytime sleepiness that they fall asleep suddenly at any time of the day, or they are "circadian-disturbed," which means that their body clocks are set so far off the "average" that it significantly interferes with their ability to function day-to-day.

If you suffer from any of these conditions, or know someone who does, read on for information and advice about the following sleep disorders:

➤ Restless Leg Syndrome or Periodic Limb Movement Disorder

➤ Sleepwalking, sleeptalking, night terrors, REM behavior disorder, bruxism

➤ Narcolepsy and circadian rhythm disorders

There's a lot to cover, so let's get started!

Twitching in the Night

Two separate conditions, Restless Leg Syndrome and Periodic Limb Movement Disorder, involve repetitive movements that disturb sleep. They represent two distinct disorders, however, each with a different set of symptoms and solutions.

As its name suggests, Restless Leg Syndrome (RLS) affects primarily the legs, although it can involve the arms as well. Practically everyone with the disorder describes the symptoms in slightly different ways, but it boils down to a "creepy-crawly," almost painful feeling in their legs that usually occurs when they're sitting or lying still. For some, RLS is very painful, but the pain is not like the kind that comes with a leg cramp or like the feeling of numbness that comes from a lack of oxygen supply to the leg. It most often involves a tingling or uncomfortable feeling in the calves that you can temporarily relieve by stretching or moving your legs.

Rest Easy

If your bed partner suffers from RLS or PLMD—or any parasomnia for that matter—you may want to sleep alone in another bed until the problem is alleviated. Otherwise, your sleep is likely to be disturbed as much or even more than that of your partner.

Although RLS occurs while you're awake, it can also affect the quantity and quality of your sleep. The constant need to stretch or move the legs to shake free of the discomfort often prevents you from falling or staying asleep. As a result, you may become sleep-deprived and suffer excessive daytime sleepiness. RLS may further interfere with your lifestyle because you may not be able to sit still for any length of time, cutting short the time you can comfortably travel or participate in other activities (such as attending a play or movie) that require sitting still.

Treatment for RLS consists of both home remedies and, in more severe and stubborn cases, drug therapy. Many sufferers find that taking a hot bath, massaging the affected leg, or applying a heating pad or ice pack to the leg helps alleviate the symptoms. Taking aspirin or other pain relievers and avoiding caffeine also may help, as can getting regular exercise. Since anemia and iron deficiency are causes of RLS, taking supplemental iron pills can help. When such home remedies fail and sleep is regularly disrupted, a doctor may prescribe a benzodiazapine (an anti-anxiety medication) or a drug commonly used to treat Parkinson's disease (L-dopa or bromocriptine, for example).

Periodic Limb Movement Disorder (PLMD), on the other hand, occurs most often when a person is fully asleep. The affected person is usually not aware of the movements, though they occur at regular intervals, usually every 30 seconds. They consist of a rhythmic extension of the big toe, together with an upward bending of the ankle, knee, or hip, each twitch lasting for one to three seconds. The movements are usually not continuous throughout the night, but instead cluster in the first half of the night during NREM sleep.

Doctors diagnose PLMD when the leg movements occur five or more times during each hour of sleep. The movements themselves appear to do no damage, and some good sleepers don't suffer from sleep deprivation or other problems because of them. However, if the twitches are strong, or if they occur in a light sleeper, they can actually wake them up. Needless to say, a main symptom of PLMD may be excessive daytime sleepiness for both those who suffer from the disorder and for their bed partners.

Unless PLMD is severe enough to disrupt your, or your partner's, sleep on a regular basis, no treatment is recommended. In some cases, doctors will prescribe the same medications used for treating RLS. Unfortunately, no home remedies have been found to alleviate the problem.

Parasomnias: Weirdness After Dark

Parasomnias are a group of conditions or behaviors that occur during, or are exacerbated by, sleep. The most common type of parasomnias are called "disorders of arousal," which include sleepwalking, sleeptalking, night terrors, and REM behavior disorder.

Experts believe the various types of arousal disorders are related and share some characteristics, including the following:

➤ Arousal usually occurs during slow-wave (Stages 3 and 4) sleep.

➤ Body movement usually takes place.

➤ Mental confusion and disorientation are present.

➤ Difficulty achieving full wakefulness occurs, along with an impaired response to external stimuli.

➤ There is difficulty recalling the episode.

These arousals generally occur when a person is in a mixed state of sleep and wakefulness, usually coming out of the deepest stages of non-dreaming sleep. Parasomnias are very common in young children, and often pass with normal development. They may persist, however, or arise for the first time later in life. Such disorders tend to run in families. Let's take a look at the different types and see what we know about why and how they occur, and what you can do to resolve them.

When Sleep Brings Terror

Night terrors (also called "sleep terrors") are the most extreme and dramatic form of arousal disorders. A night terror episode usually begins with a bloodcurdling scream or shout. Individuals experiencing night terrors have been known to bolt out of bed, to run out of the house, even to do harm to themselves or others. Their pupils are dilated, they're sweating profusely, their heart rates are elevated, and they're generally terrified. Unlike nightmares, however, night terrors occur without dream recall—those who experience them have no idea what frightens them so terribly. Sometimes the sleeper wakes without any memory at all of having been frightened or of screaming. Needless to say, night terrors are most disturbing for both those who experience them and for their bed partners and housemates.

In most cases of arousal disorders in children, there's no need to worry or even to consult a doctor. However, contact your doctor if your child experiences disturbed sleep that causes:

➤ Potentially dangerous behavior that is violent or may result in injury

➤ Extreme disturbance to other household members

➤ Excessive sleepiness during the day

No one knows what causes night terrors, although a disruption in the nervous system appears to be involved. As is true for other parasomnias, night terrors are fairly common in children, especially those between the ages of five and seven. Kids tend to outgrow the problem naturally, without treatment. Only about 1 percent of adults develop this disorder. In susceptible people, stress, sleep deprivation, or even just sleeping in a strange bed can trigger an episode of night terrors. Medication, regular exercise, and adequate sleep are the most common treatments for night terrors in adults.

Somnabilism: Up and About in the Night

Although most common in children between the ages of six and 12, sleepwalking can also plague adults. In fact, according to the American Medical Association, some four million Americans have sought help for sleepwalking, also known as somnambulism. Sleepwalking usually takes place in the first third of the night and most often involves simple walking or other repetitive movement. Remarkably, a sleepwalker is often able to safely negotiate around objects and furniture.

Usually, the episodes last only a few minutes before the individual returns to normal sleep. It is usually best not to try to wake sleepwalkers; instead, simply help them back to bed and let them wake up on their own. Nightmares, bed-wetting, and night terrors can also occur in those who sleepwalk, especially children. Interestingly enough, an EEG of a person sleepwalking shows a mixture of sleep and wake activity—in other words, a sleepwalker truly is half asleep and half awake.

Set Your Alarm!

Although it's unlikely that you'll do anything to hurt yourself or others while sleepwalking, you could fall down a flight of stairs or walk outside into traffic. To avoid such danger, sleep on the first floor, keep all doors locked, and hide the keys to the car!

Fever, sleep deprivation, or emotional upset can trigger sleepwalking. If you or your partner sleepwalks, it's important for you to seek medical advice. No one knows exactly what causes sleepwalking, but extreme stress, worry, and—rarely—a brain disorder like epilepsy may cause the disturbance. In some cases, medication like Valium, Tofranil, and even some stimulants have helped to alleviate sleepwalking.

Action After Dark

As you may remember from Chapter 2, your muscles become virtually paralyzed when you enter REM sleep— the stage of sleep in which you dream. This is a good thing, for otherwise we'd all be acting out our dreams in the middle of the night, without being conscious of our behavior.

Unfortunately, for some people, that's exactly what happens. For reasons as yet poorly understood, people who suffer from *REM behavior disorder* (RBD)—mostly older males—truly act out their dreams. In one case, reported by

Dr. James Maas in his book *Power Sleep* (Villard, 1998), a British man shot his new bride to death while he dreamt of being pursued by gangsters. According the *Encyclopedia of Sleep and Dreaming,* people with RBD do not act out "normal" dreams, but instead carry out distinctly abnormal and often violent dreams. Interestingly enough, they are rarely the aggressor in these dreams, but instead are acting out their efforts to protect themselves or their loved ones from danger.

Words to Sleep By

REM behavior disorder (RBD) is a parasomnia in which you act out part of a dream. Thought to be due to a malfunction in the brain stem cells that normally inhibit all muscle tone in REM sleep, this disorder can result in bizarre and disruptive behavior.

Indeed, RBD is a serious medical problem that can result in injury and death if left untreated. Over 75 percent of RBD patients have sustained repeated injuries such as bruises, lacerations requiring stitches, and fractures. Their bed partners are almost equally at risk—one woman, for instance, sustained three broken ribs from a single punch delivered by her sleeping husband.

No one knows what causes REM behavior disorder, but it appears that the muscles never receive the "paralysis" message from the cluster of cells in the brain stem responsible for this function. Doctors treat REM behavior disorder with medications such as clonazepam (Klonopin), a tranquilizer that is part of the class of drugs known as benzodiazepines.

The Buzz About Bruxism

No one who has ever heard it will ever forget the sound made by teeth as they grind together—the raw edge of it, the spine-tingling, nerve-shattering rasp of it. An estimated one in 20 adults and three in 20 children unconsciously grind their teeth, disturbing those around them and putting themselves at risk for serious dental trouble.

Bruxism, the grinding of teeth during sleep, is a very common occurrence and usually isn't associated with any significant medical or psychological problems. However, severe bruxism may be associated with sleep disruption and sleep deprivation. In addition, nocturnal grinding can exert thousands of pounds of pressure per square inch on teeth surfaces. It not only can damage the teeth, but also the bone, the gums, and the jaw joint.

Until recently, doctors attributed bruxism to the release of tension from emotional stress. However, many dental authorities today believe the cause is related to an unconscious effort to correct irregularities of the chewing surfaces of the teeth. Dentists term such irregularities malocclusions. Simply put, people who grind their teeth may be doing so in order to find a comfortable place to fit the upper and lower teeth together.

If you or someone you love has this nightly grind problem, your first stop should be your dentist's office. The dentist may recommend using a plastic device (mouth guard); although a mouth guard does not reduce the amount of grinding, it can be quite helpful in preventing damage to the teeth. It also mutes the grinding sound that could be disturbing your or your partner's sleep.

What Is Narcolepsy?

No doubt there have been days when you've felt so tired that it feels like you could fall asleep standing up—everybody has felt like this at some point or another.

However, in some cases, such a condition is chronic and debilitating. Called *narcolepsy,* this condition affects approximately one in 1,000 people in the United States, just about the same number affected by multiple sclerosis or Parkinson's disease. According to the National Sleep Foundation, about 250,000 Americans suffer from narcolepsy.

Defining Narcolepsy

The word *narcolepsy* comes from the Greek *narke,* for "numbness," and *lambanein,* which means "to seize." Narcolepsy is a neurological sleep disorder that essentially involves an attack of REM sleep—the dreaming portion of sleep—during the day. It is characterized by excessive daytime sleepiness, cataplexy, sleep paralysis, and hypnagogic hallucinations—terms we'll explain in more detail later in this chapter.

Words to Sleep By

Narcolepsy is a neurological sleep disorder that causes irresistible sleepiness during the day.

Narcolepsy can begin at any age and often continues throughout life. It often becomes noticeable during the teens or early twenties, but can also first appear later in life. There also seems to be genetic connection: Close relatives of people with narcolepsy are 60 times more likely to suffer from the disorder than are members of the general population.

A person with narcolepsy has recurring episodes of lapses into sleep that can last anywhere from several seconds to 10 to 20 minutes. You wake up from this "nap" feeling refreshed for an hour or two until drowsiness returns.

Called "sleep attacks," these sudden sleep episodes can occur in awkward and even dangerous situations, and often without warning.

As you may remember from Chapter 2, REM sleep begins after you've passed through the first four stages of sleep. With narcolepsy, REM sleep starts almost immediately. Since the brain may not be totally asleep when dreaming begins, the dream is sometimes experienced more vividly and is thought of as a hallucination. These REM periods, or fragments of them, occur inappropriately during the day.

The exact cause of narcolepsy is not clearly understood. It appears to be a biological problem, possibly involving abnormalities of brain chemistry. It often runs in families; geneticists have found a remarkable association between narcolepsy and the presence of a specific group of genes called *HLA-DR2*.

The Symptoms

The symptoms of narcolepsy are usually first noticed during teenage or young adult years, although it can strike at any age. Different individuals experience wide variations in both the development, the number, and the severity of their symptoms. The primary symptoms of narcolepsy include:

➤ **Excessive daytime sleepiness, often so severe that the sufferer falls asleep unexpectedly many times a day.** Persistent drowsiness that may continue for prolonged periods of time and microsleeps—fleeting moments of sleep intruding into the waking state—may also occur. Not only is this condition embarrassing, it can also be very dangerous.

➤ **Muscle weakness when emotions are strong.** Called *cataplexy*, this symptom involves sudden loss of muscle function ranging from slight weakness (such as limpness of the neck or knees, sagging facial muscles, or an inability to speak clearly) to complete body collapse. The person remains conscious throughout the episode, which may last from a few seconds to several minutes. One of the most striking features of cataplexy is its association with specific situations or emotions. The most common triggers are laughter, anger, surprise, and excitement.

Words to Sleep By

A symptom of narcolepsy, **cataplexy** is the sudden attack of complete or partial muscular paralysis, often precipitated by a strong emotion.

➤ **Inability to move for several minutes after waking up.** Called sleep paralysis (we first described this in Chapter 2), this problem is related to the disruption of REM sleep.

➤ **Vivid, realistic, often frightening dreams.** Also called hypnagogic hallucinations, these intense experiences occur at the beginning or end of the sleep period. Often the person has the sensation of being paralyzed and then perceives some threatening figure or event nearby.

The Diagnosis

If your doctor suspects narcolepsy based on a description of your symptoms, he or she will probably suggest that you visit a sleep laboratory for an evaluation. There, you'll be hooked up to a polysomnograph to measure your sleep patterns during the day and during the night. A diagnosis of narcolepsy is made if the polysomnograph shows both of the following:

➤ Falling asleep in under 10 minutes twice during the day.

➤ REM sleep occurring in less than 20 minutes.

Stay-Awake Solutions

The goal of treatment for narcolepsy is to keep you as alert as possible during the day and to minimize any recurring episodes of cataplexy. Your doctor will probably recommend one or more of the following treatments:

➤ **Medication.** The main treatment of excessive daytime sleepiness in narcolepsy is with a group of drugs called central nervous system stimulants including dextroamphetamine sulfate (Dexedrine) and methylphenidate hydrocholoride (Ritalin). For cataplexy and other REM-sleep symptoms, antidepressant medication and other drugs that suppress REM sleep are prescribed.

➤ **Scheduled naps.** An important part of treatment is scheduled short naps of about 10 to 15 minutes each, two to three times a day. Such naps help to control daytime sleepiness and keep you as alert as possible.

➤ **Avoidance of alcohol.** As you know from past chapters, drinking alcohol can disrupt your sleep—and that's just as true for those who suffer from narcolepsy.

Narcolepsy is one kind of sleep disorder that has you sleeping when you'd rather be awake. Those who suffer from circadian rhythm disorders find themselves in the same situation, though these conditions have very different symptoms, causes, and treatments.

Lark Songs and Owl Hoots

For a small percentage of the population, there is a mis-
alignment between their internal clocks and the "normal"
sleep/wake pattern followed by most of society. In other
words, they have biological clocks that keep them awake
and put them to sleep at times that are extremely disruptive to their lives. In some cases, they fall asleep and get
up way too early; in others, they go to bed and get up way
too late.

DSPS: The Late Show

Delayed Sleep Phase Syndrome (DSPS) is a fairly common
disorder of sleep timing. People with DSPS tend to fall
asleep at very late times, and also have difficulty waking
up in time for normal work, school, or social needs. Typically, the affected person is unable to fall asleep until 3 or
4 a.m. or later and finds it difficult or impossible to sustain alertness during the day if they have to wake before
10 or 11 a.m. If they are forced to rise at 7 a.m. or so to
go to a 9-to-5 job or to school, they become seriously
sleep-deprived—but even then cannot fall asleep until 3
or 4 a.m.

Because body temperature and other circadian rhythms
also tend to "run late" in people with DSPS, it is likely
that the disorder results from an abnormality in the timing mechanism that governs sleep and wakefulness. In
some cases, it could be that these people are not as sensitive to light cues as others, and therefore cannot depend
on the prime Zeitgeber of sunlight to maintain their internal clocks. In others, their natural body clocks may run
with a cycle of longer than 25 hours, causing a delay in
the onset of normal sleep periods.

The disorder often first appears in late childhood and
adolescence. In fact, some studies indicate that as

many as 15 to 20 percent of university students may be affected, though their symptoms tend to be discounted as simply a side-effect of puberty. Once established, the condition often persists for many years and may be more severe in the autumn and winter months. Unfortunately, there are some who suffer from DSPS, but never receive a proper diagnosis. These people usually blame themselves—or their families blame them—thinking that they're simply lazy and unmotivated. To counter this assumption, those with DSPS often force themselves to get up on time, by the use of multiple alarm clocks if necessary, and then struggle through the day on only two or three hours of sleep. Despite their exhaustion, however, they are often unable to fall asleep before the wee hours of the morning.

Rest Easy

It is very important to determine if your teenager's inability to get up in the morning and stay awake and alert at school results from normal changes in sleep patterns, a clinical sleep disorder like DSPS, or is related to depression or another problem, such as a learning disability. Talk to your doctor if you have concerns.

Needless to say, those with DSPS are likely to gravitate toward the night shift or to occupations with late working hours (the restaurant and entertainment industries, for instance) or flexible ones (self-employed writers, free-lance computer programmers, etc.). They are the direct opposites of their extreme Lark counterparts who suffer from a disorder called Advanced Sleep Phase Syndrome (ASPS).

ASPS: The Way-Too Early Bird

Far less common than DSPS, ASPS is a disorder in which the major sleep episode is advanced in relation to the desired clock time. This mistiming results in symptoms of compelling evening sleepiness, an early sleep onset, and an awakening that is earlier than desired, often before dawn. Typically, sleep onset occurs between 6 p.m. and 9 p.m. and wake-up before 5 a.m., sometimes as early as 1 a.m.—making those with ASPS the worst dinner dates imaginable!

In contrast to DSPS, with which teenagers and young adults are most affected, ASPS most frequently affects middle-aged and older people. In fact, as we'll discuss further in Chapter 13, early awakening is a normal part of the aging process, and ASPS may represent an extreme expression of this tendency. Like their counterparts, those with ASPS get a normal quantity and quality of sleep—when they're able to set their own schedules. Otherwise, they often become sleep-deprived as they go without sleep in order to live in the "real" world.

Resetting Your Clock

Both DSPS and ASPS respond well to two often-related treatments. The first is chronotherapy, in which—with help from experts at a sleep lab or on their own with guidance—the patients force themselves to go to bed a few hours later (in the case of DSPS) or earlier (in the case of ASPS) every day until they achieve their desired bedtime by progressively moving sleep time around the clock. This process can take up to two weeks, but is often successful. The trick, however, is that once they achieve this new, acceptable bedtime, they must NEVER deviate from it, or they'll have to start the resetting process all over again. Remember, DSPS and ASPS are disorders of the internal clock, a clock that clearly runs on its own time.

One particularly helpful adjunct to chronotherapy is bright light therapy, which we discussed in some depth in Chapter 6. Those with DSPS can move their biological clocks forward by exposing themselves to daylight first thing in the morning and avoiding bright light in the evening. People with ASPS reset their internal clocks by exposing themselves to bright light during the late evening hours and making sure to keep their bedrooms pitch black during the early morning hours. Adding a dose of melatonin, a hormone that helps set the stage for sleep, an hour or two before the appropriate bedtime can also help both types of sleep-disordered people reset their body clocks and get a good night's sleep.

Solutions for a Better Tomorrow

In almost all cases of sleep disorders and parasomnias, the better you sleep, and the less sleep-deprived you are, the less likely you'll be to suffer their symptoms. That means examining your dietary habits, reducing caffeine intake, staying away from too much alcohol before bedtime, exercising regularly, finding ways to reduce and relieve stress, and creating a sleep-friendly environment in your bedroom.

In the next chapter, we'll talk about another kind of sleep problem that stems from an external rather than internal cause: jet lag.

The Time Zone Rhumba

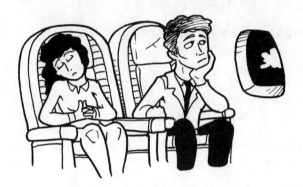

What could be more exciting and stimulating to the body, mind, and spirit than hopping on a plane, flying thousands of miles through clear blue ozone, and then arriving in a completely different landscape and environment? It still seems almost magical to us naturally earthbound humans, and the pleasure and stimulation of travel would well be worth the expense and inconvenience, if only—if only!—it weren't for the jet lag, that sickly, tired, out-of-sorts feeling that overwhelms so many people as they try to adjust to a new time and place.

Fortunately, because of all that's known about the internal circadian clock, we can help you alleviate the symptoms of jet lag on your next long-distance journey, whether it's for business or pleasure. Unless you're particularly hardy and a little bit lucky, you probably won't be able to eliminate jet lag entirely, but with some planning and extra care, you can make your time away from home a lot more comfortable.

Jet Lag: The Malady of Our Time

It seems like a cruel trick, doesn't it? There you are, the sun shining as you munch on a croissant on the Champs Élysées in Paris or as you face potential new clients at a business meeting in Toyko—and all you can think about is getting back to bed. Maybe more sleep will stop your head from throbbing, soothe your frazzled nerves, and help you remember the name of your key contact at the meeting.

And sleep would indeed help to cure your symptoms—at least in the short term. But if you were planning to spend several days or a few weeks in this new land, you'd be best served by timing your sleep very carefully right from the start. By doing so, you'd stand a better chance that— sooner rather than later—your body would catch up with the environment.

Causes and Effects of Jet Lag

If you've traveled across more than a few time zones, you already know the symptoms of the condition commonly known as jet lag. They include, among others:

➤ Headache

➤ Irritability

➤ Gastric discomfort

➤ Chills

➤ Difficulty with concentration

➤ Sleep problems

What you might not realize is that several different travel-related factors contribute to the development of these symptoms. Understanding each of them, and how they combine to make you feel just plain icky, may help protect you against their effects the next time you travel—and we'll give you tips on how to do so later in this chapter. In the meantime, it's important that you gain an understanding of just what might cause these symptoms in the first place. Among the factors influencing the development of jet lag are:

➤ **Travel fatigue.** If you've ever had to pack, get to the airport, pass through security, stand in line to check your luggage, and then wait at the stuffy gate before cramming onto a tiny, overcrowded airplane, you know just what we mean by "travel fatigue." By the time you arrive at your destination, you're more than ready for a long night's sleep in order to recover. As you'll see later, if you time it right, this state of exhaustion can actually help you in the long run.

➤ **Sleep loss.** Unless you're one of the lucky few who find it possible—even easy—to sleep on a plane, or unless your entire flight takes place during your normal daytime, you're bound to leave the plane running a sleep deficit. Again, if you're able to time your flight optimally, such a condition may work to your advantage.

➤ **External desynchronization.** You exit the plane ready for breakfast, but it's dinnertime at your new location. It's dark outside, the traffic is sparse, the shades are drawn across apartment windows, no birds are chirping in the sun, and the daily newspaper won't be delivered for another several hours. You feel disjointed somehow, a little confused and unsettled, and these feelings only progress after you arrive at the hotel and try to sleep when your body urges you to stay awake. This feeling of being out-of-synch with your environment is itself a symptom of jet lag.

Words to Sleep By

Desynchronization is the disruption of a set pattern of events or processes that normally are coordinated. With jet lag, many different biological functions normally synchronized by the internal body clock become disrupted.

➤ **Internal desynchronization.** In addition to feeling "dislocated" because your sense of what time it is differs from the real time in your new location, you also have to cope with a very interesting and little-known side effect of time-zone travel: internal desynchronization, the disruption of your carefully orchestrated biological rhythms. The foremost casualty is, of course, your sleep/wake cycle. Not only may your body be telling you to stay awake during local nighttime, but anxiety, stress, fatigue, and excitement all act together to further disrupt this cycle. Many travelers, for instance, spend less time in the restorative Stages 3 and 4 and REM sleep. They also have more trouble getting to and staying asleep—no matter what time it is locally or internally. In addition, as you may remember from Chapter 1, many of your physiological functions, such as your blood pressure and body temperature, have their own daily rhythms, which are kept in synch by your internal clock. With time-zone travel, all these rhythms become desynchronized, one from the other, which contributes to your feelings of malaise. Constipation and other symptoms of gastrointestinal distress, headaches, and irritability are just a few of the resulting symptoms. It can take several days for your body rhythms to readjust and run smoothly and in harmony with your new environment.

Go East, Go West

As you may have experienced yourself, the direction of the flight you take significantly influences the degree of jet lag you experience. When you fly eastbound, or against the direction of the sun, jet lag tends to be more severe than when you fly west. That's because when flying westward, you're allowing your body to follow its natural inclination to extend the day to 25 hours. Your bedtime shifts later and later. Let's say you're a New Yorker and you travel to Los Angeles. Within three days, without even trying, your bedtime would quickly shift so that you're going to bed at the same time as your Angeleno counterparts.

By traveling east, on the other hand, you're forcing your body to go against the natural tendency. If you're from San Francisco and travel to Boston, for example, your body will want to keep awake and active (in effect, to extend the day) but, in order to catch up, you'd be best served by going to bed earlier than your body might prefer.

A study of the 1991, 1992, and 1993 records for 19 major-league baseball teams in the Eastern and Pacific time zones of North America shows just how dramatic the difference can be between eastward and westward travel. Those teams that traveled west to east tended to lose the games they played away far more often than those that traveled east to west. The home team won 56 percent of the games, said the researchers, but the probability of winning depended on whether the visiting team had just traveled eastward.

Rest Easy

If you're an Owl, you'll probably fare better than Larks when flying west. That's because you naturally want to stay up very late into the night and get up quite late in the day, which helps you advance your sleep/wake patterns. If you're a Lark, eastward travel is better for you, because you find it easier to get up earlier in the morning than to shift to a later bedtime.

Nevertheless, no matter which way you're traveling, for how long, or how far, you're bound to feel some ill effects. The only exception is north-south destinations. Indeed, flying north to south—say from Chicago to Rio de Janeiro—is not nearly as disruptive as east-west travel. That's because you don't have to adjust to a vastly differ-ent time zone. However, you will suffer from other side effects: fatigue, sleep loss, and symptoms of air travel such as dehydration and irritability.

You can help minimize the effects of jet lag in two ways: by preparing well for your journey ahead of time and by working to readjust your biological clock as efficiently as possible.

Prevention Is the Best Cure

Although for most people it's impossible to eliminate all the negative effects of travel on the body and mind, you can help minimize them by being as healthy and well-rested as possible before you get on the plane and by treating yourself well during the flight. Here are a few tips to get you started:

> ➤ **Get plenty of sleep *before* you travel.** The effects of jet lag are considerably greater if you're already carrying a sleep debt when you travel. Not only will you feel the symptoms of sleep deprivation—excessive daytime sleepiness, headaches, irritability, and so on—but lack of sleep will also exacerbate the disruption of your circadian rhythms.

> ➤ **Try a gradual approach pre-flight.** If you're traveling west and have some flexibility with your routine, you can try going to bed and getting up an hour later each day for three days before leaving—that way, you'll be well on your way to meeting the local schedule by the time you arrive. If you're flying eastward, you'll want to reverse the process by going to bed and getting up an hour earlier each day.

> ➤ **Avoid dehydration.** Airplane travel is highly conducive to dehydration because the air is so dry in the cabin. Dehydration results in diminished blood flow to the muscles, reduced kidney function, and fatigue, all of which exacerbate jet lag. You can prevent dehydration by drinking one liter of water for every six hours of flight time, even if you don't feel thirsty.

> ➤ **Avoid alcohol.** Alcohol not only affects the quality of your sleep, but also tends to dehydrate the body, two effects you want to avoid if you're trying to alleviate jet lag.

> ➤ **Exercise.** Although you can't play tennis on board, you certainly can stretch, walk up and down the aisle, and even perform some isometric exercises in your seat. Doing so will help keep your body limber and reduce stress during a long flight.

➤ **Be prepared for sleep on the plane.** In addition to timing your sleep period carefully, you also want to come aboard prepared to improve your sleep environment. Earplugs, an eye mask, an inflatable neck pillow, and a sweater or shawl will help make you more comfortable, and thus more likely to relax and fall asleep.

Set Your Alarm!

Don't wait to grab an airline pillow and blanket. By the time you need to take a nap, more seasoned and adept travelers will have nabbed them all for themselves.

➤ **Eat well.** Generally speaking, it's best to eat several small, light meals throughout the days before, during, and just following your journey. Eating a big, heavy meal will only increase your chances of suffering an upset stomach. Avoid high-sugar snacks, caffeine, and alcohol, all of which can interfere with your ability to sleep and make you feel uncomfortable. Needless to say, airline food is NOT necessarily the best choice for you. We suggest you pack your own healthful "mini-meals" and forgo the on-line service.

On the Road with Your Internal Clock

In addition to making it through your journey feeling healthy and vital, you'll also want to speed the rate at which your internal clock adjusts to the time in your new environment. No matter what you do, this process is apt to take at least a couple of days. Of course, the more quickly and deeply you can fall asleep at local bedtime and wake up feeling rested in the morning, the better. Here are some tips to help you do just that:

➤ **Choose your strategy.** Your very first decision when it comes to your biological clock is whether or not you want to stay on your "home time" or make the adjustment to your new environment. To a large extent, that decision depends on how long you're planning to stay at your travel destination: If it's a very short trip—less than three days—and you have control over your time (you're on vacation, for example), you may be best served by maintaining your home schedule as much as possible. If you're staying longer, or have business meetings to attend that require you to be alert when you'd be sleepy at home, you'll want to readjust your circadian clock as soon as you can.

➤ **Schedule your trip with care.** The best itinerary has you arriving at your destination in the early evening (local time). That way, you'll be able to get a light bite to eat, take a walk to work out the kinks, and have a little time to relax before hitting the sack. Because you'll already be tired from the sheer act of traveling, you may be tired enough to sleep even if it's earlier than usual on "body time." If not, see the information that's coming up on melatonin and light.

➤ **Anticipate your new time zone.** If you're flying when it's nighttime at your destination and it'll be morning when you arrive, try to sleep on the plane. If it's daytime, try to stay awake—no matter what time your body thinks it is at the moment—or at most catch a 20-minute power nap to take the edge off.

➤ **Time your light exposure.** And no, we don't mean for your camera—we mean your body's exposure to light, especially sunlight. Indeed, light therapy can be very helpful in resetting your internal clock, as long as you're careful about when and how long to expose yourself to it. As you may remember from Chapter 6—and we suggest you reread that chapter if you're confused about how light affects your biological clock—exposure to bright light in the morning will help shift you forward, allowing you to go to bed earlier and wake up earlier in the coming days. Bright light in the evening, on the other hand, will shift you back, so that you're going to bed later and getting up later. Combined with taking a dose of melatonin about an hour or so before bedtime, bright-light therapy can significantly speed up your period of adjustment to a new environment.

Rest Easy

If you intend to stay less than three days in a new time zone, you can avoid most symptoms of travel-related malaise by simply sticking to your "home" schedule as closely as possible. For example, if you're a Bostonian who flies to London for an afternoon business meeting and only intend to stay one night, time your major sleep period to coincide with Boston rather than London time.

➤ **Use melatonin wisely.** Taking a dose of melatonin before you want to go to bed at your destination may help set the stage for your body to sleep, even if it's daytime back home. DO NOT take melatonin before this point—if you do, you may end up disturbing your rhythms unnecessarily.

➤ **Avoid using sleeping pills.** Although a quick fix for a travel-related sleep problem may seem like a dream come true (literally!), in the end, you'll probably only make things worse for yourself. The "hangover" effect of most sleeping pills will only increase your feelings of sleep deprivation the next day, and may even make it harder for you to get to sleep the next night.

➤ **Make the most of your hotel.** When you book your hotel, find out what kinds of "jet-lag treatment" services they offer. Some hotels offer rooms equipped with black-out curtains that allow you to sleep even when the sun is shining brightly outside, full-spectrum light sources if you require more light to reset your clock and it's still dark outside, and room service that can prepare whatever meal your body clock desires (dinner at 7 a.m. if need be).

➤ **Nap wisely.** As discussed in Chapter 8, napping can be a godsend when it comes to making up for sleep loss or preparing the body for a good night's sleep by taking the edge off exhaustion. Once again, though, timing is everything. You'll want to keep your naps short, from 10 to 30 minutes, and avoid napping within four to five hours of local bedtime.

There's new evidence that the world is getting smaller every day—but your body doesn't necessarily agree! Armed with the advice in this chapter, however, you should be able to improve your chances of having a healthy, happy journey the next time you join the jet set.

Chapter 12

Pulling All-Nighters

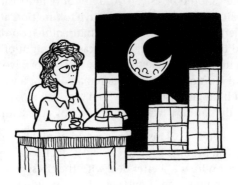

In This Chapter

➤ The world of night work

➤ Understanding the effects of working nights

➤ Learning to make the best of a tough work schedule

A 24-hour society. . .that's pretty much the state of the world as we speed headlong into the 21st century. There are fast becoming very few limits to the activities we can perform at any hour of the day almost anywhere in the world.

For millions of years, however, our ancestors awakened with the sun and slept after dark. Because of our intrinsic, biological need for sleep at night, most of us still go to bed around 11 p.m. and get up by 7 a.m. (give or take an hour or two at each end). We prefer to sleep at this time because our bodies are primed to do so by the internal time-keeper known as the biological clock.

But things are different for the 20 million Americans who work the night shift and the millions who provide care for loved ones who need attention around the clock. These people must resist their natural instincts and stay up when they should be asleep. And not only must they simply remain awake, but they also have to function at high levels, performing sensitive tasks that require coordination and thought. Although an occasional night of sleeplessness may cause some temporary discomfort, working the night shift over the long haul may disrupt a wide range of biological rhythms, which can lead to a variety of potentially serious psychological and physical symptoms.

In this chapter, we'll discuss the world of night work and the physical problems it can cause. We'll also offer you some tips on how to better deal with the stress that night work puts on your body and soul. First, we'll help you get through the night when you're feeling sleep-deprived, then we'll show you how to manage over the long haul with tips on how to improve your general health habits and get as much sleep as possible on a regular basis.

The Hazards of Shift Work

It's important to know right from the start that, unless you're one of the lucky few extreme Owls who naturally thrive at night or you learn to reset your biological clock by judicious use of light and other methods, your body simply won't "get used" to working when it otherwise would be sleeping.

At the very least, the side effects of working at night are uncomfortable. They not only can have a negative impact on your general health, they can also disrupt your family and social life. The level of disruption night work causes depends both on how flexible your body is to changes in schedule and the type of shift you work. In fact, there are several types of shift work schedules—rotating shifts; fixed 8, 10, and 12-hour shifts; evening shifts; night shifts; and thousands of variations of these shifts—each with its own set of advantages, disadvantages, and side effects. Because it goes far beyond the scope of this book to discuss specifics of each shift work type, we'll focus on some of the most common and more general problems caused by working at night on a regular basis.

Before we get started, we do want to reiterate that some people actually thrive on the night shift. Natural Owls, for instance, find themselves attracted to this lifestyle because it suits their innate tendency to function best at night. Some Regular Robins can adapt easily and well to working at night, and also enjoy the freedom of having the afternoons off that such a schedule permits.

Rest Easy

To find out how well you'd adapt to shift work, ask yourself how long you can sleep during the day after an "all-nighter." If you can sleep for seven or eight hours, you may do well. Then ask yourself how well you handle jet lag. The ability to bounce back from a six-hour time change within a day or two indicates that you may be a good candidate for shift work.

Nevertheless, many night workers find themselves plagued with symptoms and side effects—medical and social—resulting from the disruption of circadian rhythms.

The Physical Effects of Night Work

As you know by now, your body has its own internal schedule, one that keeps you alert and awake during the day and asleep at night. Whenever you disrupt this rhythm—due to jet lag, night work, or a sleep disorder—you risk developing some related medical problems, some minor, others more serious. Here are some of the most common:

➤ **Mood and memory problems.** Just one night of missed sleep can make you cranky and forgetful, so you can imagine what running at a near-constant sleep debt does to your psychological stability! In addition, a few studies suggest that shift work may be linked to depression. A study of Italian textile workers, for instance, found that night workers reported a far higher incidence of anxiety or depression requiring treatment than day workers.

➤ **Sleep deprivation.** Over time, the average night worker obtains about two hours less sleep a day than the average nine-to-fiver. One study reported that between one- and two-thirds of night workers report that they fall asleep at least once a week on the job. In addition, according to the American Sleep Disorders Association, five million people suffer from sleep deprivation as a result of shift work.

➤ **Possible increased risk of infection.** A 1996 study in the *Journal of Experimental Biology* found that people forced to stay up later than usual showed a decrease in the activity of *natural killer cells,* immune system blood cells that fight disease.

Words to Sleep By

Natural killer cells, often abbreviated NK, are immune system cells that form a line of defense against infection. When you lose sleep, your body fails to produce its usual supply of these cells, which could leave you more vulnerable to infection.

➤ **Gastrointestinal disorders.** Numerous studies show that working nights raises an employee's risk of developing a variety of gastrointestinal problems, including ulcers, bowel irregularities (constipation or diarrhea), excessive gas, abdominal pain, and heartburn. Shift work is hard on the stomach for a number of reasons that include lack of sleep, disruption of circadian rhythms, poor eating habits, excessive coffee and alcohol consumption, smoking, and stress.

➤ **Cardiovascular disease.** The general consensus is that shift work raises an individual's risk of developing heart disease by 30 to 50 percent, even after accounting for lifestyle factors such as smoking and diet. That makes it less of a risk than smoking cigarettes or being obese, for instance, but still a significant problem. The connection between shift work and heart disease may involve several factors. The disruption to circadian rhythms may increase blood pressure and blood cholesterol levels, both of which contribute to the development of heart disease. The high stress levels experienced by shift workers also add to the risk. In addition, studies show that shift workers are more likely than day workers to lead sedentary lives, be overweight, and consume high-fat diets, all risk factors for heart disease.

➤ **Reproductive risks.** Some studies suggest that shift work can affect a woman's ability to get pregnant and carry a fetus to term. A European study, for instance, found that women shift workers on rotating schedules experience conception delays of more than nine months when they try to conceive. A British study found that shift work increased the risk of miscarriage by 44 percent, while a French study found that shift work increased the risk of premature births by 60 percent.

As startling as these statistics are, it's important to keep them in perspective. First, just because there is an increased risk across the population doesn't mean that you as an individual will suffer such an increase. Second, shift work ranks near the bottom of the list of avoidable risk factors: Smoking, obesity, and lack of exercise are far more important in the development of heart disease, for instance, than shift work. Finally, there is still much to be learned about the effects of shift work on health, and the conclusions reached in the studies we cite here may or may not be modified as we learn more.

Equally variable are the effects of shift work on family relationships. Some families adjust quite well, especially if they structure their time wisely and plan family activities with care. Others have more difficulty, as you'll see in the next section.

The Impact of Shift Work on Family Life

As practically any American adult can tell you today, balancing work and family life is a demanding responsibility even under the best of circumstances. Add to it the challenges posed by shift work, and you may have a recipe for familial discord and miscommunication. In fact, studies show the divorce rate in shift-working families is 60 percent higher than for day workers. Indeed, the stresses on family life when one or both parents work around the clock or have irregular schedules are great:

➤ **The absent parent.** Needless to say, shift work makes it more difficult than ever to spend time with your children. The evening shift (usually 4 p.m. to midnight) may be the toughest, since you leave for work before your children return from school and get home after they're in bed. And if you and your spouse both work shifts, the chances that your children will get all the attention they need from you are even more remote.

➤ **Family stress.** You're tired and cranky when you get home from a 12-hour shift, but your spouse and children crave your attention. Instead of giving it to them, you crawl into bed and throw the covers over your head for hours. When you wake up, the last thing you want to do is fix a family meal or repair the broken lawn mower (which you promised to do a week ago). Resentment can build, and build quickly, among all family members.

As you can see, working nights can disrupt many aspects of your life if you're not careful. Later in the chapter, we'll offer some tips on how to make the best of your time off, including how to get the sleep you need to protect your health as much as possible.

Rest Easy

Check out Circadian Technologies' Web site at www.circadian.com. This site is filled with information about circadian rhythms, sleep deprivation and its effects, and how to better cope with shift work physically, mentally, and socially. The site also offers a variety of pamphlets, booklets, newsletters, and other material for shift workers and their managers.

In the meantime, let's discuss another challenge for many people who work the night shift: making it through the long nights awake and alert when your body craves sleep.

Staying Up and Alert

With any luck, you'll be one of the few who adapt well to shift work, which means that you'll be able to get the sleep you need during the day and thus avoid becoming sleep-deprived. Even so, you may have trouble making it through the entire night without experiencing a dip in energy and concentration at some point during your shift, particularly in the early morning hours.

In Chapter 8, we outlined some of the ways you can help your body feel more alert and focused—suggestions that certainly bear repeating here. We've also added a few others more specifically targeted to the shift worker, including:

➤ **Come to work rested.** We know that's easier said than done, which is why we'll give you some tips on how to sleep during the day later in the chapter. But simply put, the more sleep you get, the better you'll be able to accommodate the demands made on your body and mind during the nights you must stay awake. Getting an uninterrupted night's sleep or learning to nap efficiently can help you maintain a proper sleep balance.

➤ **Vary your tasks.** If possible, take a break from the more repetitive tasks involved in your job and turn to ones that require either more intellectual creativity or more physical energy. The change in pace, along with the new demand on your attention, will help wake you up.

➤ **Take an exercise break.** Even a short burst of exercise can help stimulate blood flow to the brain and your extremities, helping you feel more alert and refreshed. Longer bouts of exercise at night can also help you shift your circadian rhythms.

➤ **Perk up.** And yes, we mean with caffeine, judiciously ingested. By timing your use of caffeine, you can make it through the most difficult hours of the night without jeopardizing your sleep during the day. Although you should avoid drinking cup after cup of coffee, tea, or cola on the night shift, one or two well-timed cups will boost your alertness when you're most tired. Keep in mind, however, that sensitivity to caffeine varies considerably from one individual to another. Depending on your physiology, a cup of coffee early in your shift may or may not interfere with sleep when you get home. If you find it does, try substituting an ice-cold glass of water or fruit juice for coffee.

Set Your Alarm!

Eating a large meal during your break will only make you feel sleepier. Try a bout of moderate exercise instead. Indeed, exercising late at night can help you adjust your circadian rhythms, theoretically making it easier to sleep in the daytime and stay awake at night.

➤ **Avoid the pharmaceutical approach.** Avoid taking pharmaceutical "uppers" or sleeping pills. Their effects on your body can be dramatic and long-lasting. They can also become addictive.

➤ **Lighten up.** In Chapter 6, we discussed the profound effects of bright light on your circadian rhythms. In addition to using light to shift your internal clock forward (or back, as the case may be), simply raising light levels in the work place can help you stay alert and suppress sleepiness.

➤ **Take a breath—of cool air.** Cool dry air, especially if it blows on your face, can help keep you awake and alert. Keep the room temperature cool as well, wearing a sweater if necessary for comfort.

Rest Easy

If you work at night, it's especially important to take care when driving. If possible, take a short nap before you leave work to take the edge off your fatigue and sleepiness. On your way home, keep the car cool and the radio on to fight fatigue—especially if you're wearing dark sunglasses to shut out morning light in order to sleep when you get home.

Making It Through Night After Night

Although most people seem to accept the fact that some of us need to work during important social functions, they have less sympathy when you're "only" trying to sleep.

Indeed, it may sometimes seem as if the entire world is out to get you. Neighbors insist on mowing their lawns while you're trying to sleep. People who would never phone you at 2 a.m. (when you might just be awake!) routinely do so at 2 p.m., not understanding that they're interrupting your major sleep period.

Many studies show that those people who are most successful at shift work don't try to live in two worlds. They install answering machines, black-out curtains, and "Do Not Disturb" signs for their bedroom doors. Their friends and family know about—and respect—the importance of uninterrupted daytime sleep.

Rest Easy

To help you organize your time and help your family remain up-to-date about your schedule, try using Circadian Technologies' *Working Nights Family Calendar.* The calendar comes with removable color-coded stickers that help everyone, including young children, understand your schedule at a glance. You can order from their Web site at www.shiftwork.com/bookstore/.

You have two basic goals here: to get enough sleep so you stay healthy while you work shifts, and to organize your time so your family and social life suffer as little as possible. Meeting those goals takes time and practice. We hope some of these tips help you get started.

Resetting Your Body Clock

Finding a way to restore your body's energy and vitality when sleep comes at strange times can be a challenge. Here are a few suggestions that might help you keep your clock running in the right direction:

➤ **Split sleeping.** This is a technique that involves sleeping for several hours immediately before and several hours immediately after a night shift. Don't concern yourself with being exact about the split: The point is to get yourself two satisfying sleep periods that total the sleep you need in any 24-hour period.

➤ **Anchor sleeping.** Anchor sleeping involves finding a time of day in which you can *always* sleep and sleeping at that time, whether you're working at night or not. Regularly taking a four-hour sleep period, say from 8 a.m. until noon, even on their days off, is one way for night workers to maintain adjustment to night work. However, this approach may be difficult to pursue if you have a rotating schedule that requires you to work some mornings during this period.

➤ **Napping.** A 90-minute nap just prior to your night shift will help you remain alert and allow for better sleep when you get home. And taking a short, 15- or 20-minute nap just before you leave work will help you avoid the hazards of drowsy driving.

➤ **Understand the power of light and dark.** Remember, the sun is an important partner in your effort to work at night and sleep during the day. If you time your exposure to light properly, you can help shift your biological clock. Basically, if you want to stay up later at night and sleep during the morning hours, avoid light in the morning by wearing dark sunglasses on your way home, then sleep in a dark room. Later, treat yourself to a burst of bright light in the late evening using a light visor or light box. Review Chapter 6 for more information about timing your light exposure to shift your rhythms and some of the high-tech (but affordable) devices that can help you do so.

Creating a Conducive Environment

Face it: Getting the sleep you need during the day is going to be a challenge because what you really want to do is create nighttime conditions—darkness, quiet, privacy, a sense of coziness—right smack in the middle of the day. Let's see what you can do to create an environment conducive to sleep despite daytime distractions:

➤ **Stay in the dark.** Black-out curtains and blinds will help keep the daylight from streaming in your windows. Keep your door closed against ambient light from the rest of the house.

Set Your Alarm!

Avoid turning on the television when you get home. The morning news and talk shows are far too perky and stimulating for someone who puts sleep as his or her top priority. Wait until later to catch up on the day's events.

➤ **Quiet please!** Noise control is essential. Unplug the telephone in your room and place the answering machine far from where you can hear it pick up incoming calls. Running an air conditioner can help mask noise from outside (as well as keep the air at a comfortably cool temperature, which will also help you sleep). Ask neighbors ahead of time if they could refrain from mowing their lawns or indulging in any other noisy activity during the hours you sleep.

➤ **Aim for comfort.** Keep your bedroom at a comfortable temperature, preferably with circulating air. Make sure your mattress and pillows support your back and head.

➤ **Establish a sleepy time routine.** Yes, it's just as important to ready your body and mind for sleep during the day as it is at night. Take a warm bath, brush your teeth, read for a little while until you feel relaxed—not exhausted, not stressed, just relaxed enough to let the pressures of your work night fade away. Then slip between the sheets and sleep.

Healthy Habits and Night Work

It's more important than ever to treat your body well: You want to be as healthy as possible to endure the extra strain working at night can impose. Here are some suggestions for staying healthy:

➤ **Get regular exercise.** And the emphasis is on "regular." Being physically fit in general will help you better withstand the rigors of night work. In addition, you can use exercise like bright light exposure or anchor sleep to help you maintain or shift your body clock. Try exercising in the late afternoon when it's still sunny out and before your next shift.

➤ **Eat well.** When you work the night shift, it may be tempting to rely on high-fat, high-sugar, quick pick-me-ups and to forget the essentials of a balanced diet. When you get home from work, it may help to eat a light meal high in carbohydrates, such as a bowl of high-fiber cereal, which will help you sleep better. For more information about how diet affects sleep, see Chapter 5.

➤ **Take time out to relax.** It's all too easy to feel as if you have to spend every waking second doing something useful. But in order to stay healthy, you also need some downtime, when you do nothing else but relax your body and soul. Watching a videotape of last Monday night's football game is one way, practicing yoga is another. Chapter 5 provides lots of hints about reducing stress in your life.

Balancing Work and Family

The challenges facing a worker on the night shift go far beyond the physical: Indeed, his or her entire circle of family and friends is often affected by the demands of, and often the unpredictability of, shift work. Here are a few suggestions to help mitigate the stress:

➤ **Share schedule information.** Make sure your family members know what your work schedule is and keep them informed about any changes that occur on a daily basis. If you're facing a permanent change—from the night shift to the evening shift, for instance—you need to discuss how this change will affect the family *before* the schedule takes effect.

➤ **Keep the lines of communication open.** Keep abreast of your family's needs so that day-to-day responsibilities, such as car maintenance or childcare, don't get lost in the shuffle. Even trivial matters can become major irritants if you ignore them for too long.

➤ **Maintain a "Family Bulletin Board."** Help everyone stay in touch by hanging up a bulletin board where you and your family can leave notes, report cards to sign, and other important messages for one another.

➤ **Plan dates for days when you're rested.** If you have trouble finding time to be alone with your partner, make a date to do something special at least once a month. When it comes to planning family outings, try to do so on days when you're likely to feel well rested, which is often not on your first day off after a week of night work. Plan carefully.

You've now read about insomnia and jet lag and shift work, and we hope you've learned enough about your own sleep problem to begin to solve it. Rest easy!

Your Sleep Log

It's important to keep track of both the quality of your sleep and your sleep-wake patterns. To help you meet that goal, we provide here a Sleep Log. We suggest you photocopy this log and save several pages of Sleep Log forms so that you can continue the process in the month and years to come.

Your Sleep Log

Date _____

Worktime _____

Playtime _____

Bedtime _____

Lights Out _____

Sleep Onset _____

Awakenings

Number/length _____

Wake-Up Time _____

Rise Time _____

Sleep Quality (1=terrible, 2=poor, 3=fair, 4=good, 5=very good, 6=excellent) _____

Nap Time/Duration _____

Date _____

Worktime _____

Playtime _____

Bedtime _____

Lights Out _____

Sleep Onset _____

Awakenings

Number/length _____

Wake-Up Time _____

Rise Time _____

Sleep Quality (1=terrible, 2=poor, 3=fair, 4=good,
5=very good, 6=excellent) _____

Nap Time/Duration _____

Date _____

Worktime _____

Playtime _____

Bedtime _____

Lights Out _____

Sleep Onset _____

Awakenings

Number/length _____

Wake-Up Time _____

Rise Time _____

Sleep Quality (1=terrible, 2=poor, 3=fair, 4=good, 5=very good, 6=excellent) _____

Nap Time/Duration _____

Date _____

Worktime _____

Playtime _____

Bedtime _____

Lights Out _____

Sleep Onset _____

Awakenings

Number/length _____

Wake-Up Time _____

Rise Time _____

Sleep Quality (1=terrible, 2=poor, 3=fair, 4=good, 5=very good, 6=excellent) _____

Nap Time/Duration _____

Date _____

Worktime _____

Playtime _____

Bedtime _____

Lights Out _____

Sleep Onset _____

Awakenings

Number/length _____

Wake-Up Time _____

Rise Time _____

Sleep Quality (1=terrible, 2=poor, 3=fair, 4=good, 5=very good, 6=excellent) _____

Nap Time/Duration _____

Date _____

Worktime _____

Playtime _____

Bedtime _____

Lights Out _____

Sleep Onset _____

Awakenings

Number/length _____

Wake-Up Time _____

Rise Time _____

Sleep Quality (1=terrible, 2=poor, 3=fair, 4=good, 5=very good, 6=excellent) _____

Nap Time/Duration _____

Glossary

Unless you've delved into the world of sleep in the past, reading this book probably opened your eyes to a variety of new concepts about sleep and body rhythms, concepts that had some words and terms you may have been unfamiliar with. We hope the following glossary of terms helps you on your journey to a good night's sleep.

Alzheimer's disease   A type of dementia; a progressive degeneration of the brain that occurs in about 5 to 10 percent of the population over the age of 65. Like many other brain disorders, Alzheimer's disease may cause sleep disturbances.

Apnea   From the Greek word *pnoia* meaning "breath" and the Greek prefix *a* denoting "absence"; apnea is the temporary cessation of breathing for any reason. Obstructive Sleep Apnea is a common sleep disorder.

Automatic behavior   A phenomenon reported by the sleep deprived in which they perform relatively routine behavior without having any memory of doing so. Automatic behavior can be quite dangerous if the behavior involves driving an automobile or performing a routine but sensitive task at work.

Autonomic nervous system   The part of the nervous system responsible for largely unconscious bodily functions such as heartbeat, blood pressure, and digestion. It is divided into two divisions, the sympathetic and parasympathetic.

Biofeedback   A behavior modification therapy in which patients are taught to control bodily functions such as blood pressure and heart rate through conscious effort.

Biofeedback can be especially helpful in learning to reduce stress.

Brain stem   The part of the nervous system located at the base of the brain, connecting the spinal cord with the rest of the brain. The brain stem contains essential mechanisms that regulate sleep/wake behavior.

Cataplexy   Sudden spell of weakness—often related to an intense emotional reaction—due to a decrease in muscle tone. Cataplexy is one of the most important symptoms of narcolepsy.

Chronobiology   The study of the biological clocks used by humans and other living things to keep time, and the biological rhythms these clocks maintain.

Chronotherapy   A specific treatment method devised to correct disruptions of circadian rhythms, particularly the sleep disorders Delayed Sleep Phase Syndrome, Advanced Sleep Phase Syndrome, and related problems.

Circadian rhythm   From the Latin *circa*, meaning "about," and *dies*, meaning "day," a circadian rhythm is a biological event that regularly recurs about every 24 hours.

Colic   A problem that occurs in infants involving long crying spells. Colic may disrupt the sleep patterns of both parent and child.

Continuous Positive Airway Pressure (CPAP)   Treatment for Obstructive Sleep Apnea that works by reversing the negative pressure that causes the throat to collapse during sleep. A machine pumps air through a plastic mask that fits over the nose. The air pressure holds the throat open, which allows for continuous breathing and prevents the frequent awakening suffered by most people with Obstructive Sleep Apnea.

Cortisol   A steroid hormone produced by the adrenal glands that affects metabolism, the stress response, and the process of inflammation. Like other hormones, cortisol is released in the body with a circadian rhythm.

Delayed Sleep Phase Disorder (DSPS)   Sleep disorder characterized by the inability to fall asleep and awaken according to ordinary schedules. Typically, the affected person is unable to fall asleep until 3 or 4 a.m. and finds it difficult to awaken earlier than 10 or 11 a.m. Once asleep, however, someone with DSPS sleeps normally.

Dementia   A term used to describe any number of conditions that involve a generalized, progressive, and usually irreversible deterioration of memory and cognition. One type of age-related dementia is Alzheimer's disease. Most, if not all, types of dementia cause sleep problems.

Depression   A mental disorder that often involves feelings of sadness and despair, but also slowed thinking, decreased pleasure, appetite changes, physical aches and pains, and sleeping difficulties.

Electroencephalograph (EEG)   A recording of the electrical signals generated by the brain; frequently used by sleep researchers to evaluate sleep patterns and identify potential sleep disorders.

Electromyogram (EMG)   A recording of the electrical signals created when muscle fibers contract. Used by sleep researchers to detect the movements associated with certain sleep stages and sleep disorders.

Electrooculograph (EOG)   A recording of eye movements during sleep.

Endogenous   A word used to describe a rhythm or condition that arises within the body and is not caused or triggered by external or environmental factors.

Entrainment   Term used by sleep researchers to describe the process by which internal biological rhythms such as sleep/wake patterns become synchronized to external Zeitgebers.

Free running   Term used in chronobiology to indicate a biological rhythm no longer synchronized with the environment.

Human growth hormone   Body chemical secreted by the pituitary gland during deep, non-REM sleep that works to promote body growth and repair.

Hypnagogic hallucination   A dream-like experience that occurs in the interval between wakefulness and sleep; common among normal sleepers, but also one of the four classic signs of narcolepsy.

Hypnic jerk   Sudden spontaneous jerk of part or all of the body that occurs during the drowsy period or during light sleep, making it difficult to fall and stay asleep.

Infradian rhythm   A biological rhythm that regularly recurs with a periodicity of longer than 24 hours.

Insomnia   The inability to fall or stay asleep at the right time, for the right length of time, and with sufficient quality to feel well and alert during the day.

Internal desynchronization   The loss of synchrony among two or more internal circadian rhythms; a frequent side effect of jet lag.

Jet lag   Maladjustment experienced when travel across time zones results in an abrupt change in the length of day. This causes body time to become out of synch with local clock time.

Lark   A person whose natural rhythms causes him or her to prefer the early morning hours for activity and concentration, and who prefers to go to bed fairly early in the evenings.

Light therapy   A procedure for treating Seasonal Affective Disorder and other disorders related to length of day, exposure to daylight, or shifts in circadian rhythms, including Delayed Phase Sleep Disorder (DSPS), Advanced Phase Disorder (ASPS), jet lag and some shift work. Involves exposure to bright light at specific times in order to shift the biological clock or to maintain rhythms that may otherwise be lost.

Melatonin   A hormone released into the bloodstream by the pineal gland, which is stimulated by darkness and prohibited by light.

Microsleep   A very brief (less than 30-second), involuntary episode of sleep that occurs during ongoing wakeful activity. A frequent symptom of extreme sleep deprivation.

Multiple Sleep Latency Test   A test used to measure how long it takes for a person to fall asleep during the day, and thus a person's daytime level of sleepiness and sleep deprivation.

Narcolepsy   A sleep disorder characterized by excessive, irresistible daytime sleepiness that causes someone to fall asleep at inappropriate times. Other symptoms include cataplexy, sleep paralysis, and hypnagogic hallucinations.

Nightmare   A frightening dream that one remembers or the experience of awakening feeling frightened. Nightmares occur during REM sleep.

Night terror   A phenomenon occurring in deep sleep in which the person is terrified and often screaming and sitting up in bed or even sleepwalking.

Night owl   Someone whose natural rhythms cause them to prefer staying up late at night and avoiding the morning hours. A night owl generally feels most alert and competent in the evening.

NREM sleep   Non-Rapid Eye Movement sleep include Stages 1–4 of the sleep cycle—all but the dreaming portion of sleep.

Obstructive Sleep Apnea   A sleep disorder involving an obstruction of the air passages, particularly the airway between the nasal openings and the voice box. Symptoms include heavy snoring, frequent awakenings, and daytime sleepiness.

Parasomnia   A disturbance during sleep such as sleepwalking, sleeptalking, bedwetting, and night terrors.

Phase response curve   A graph describing the resetting of the timing of a circadian rhythm by a Zeitgeber, and how the shift varies in direction and length according to the time of day that the Zeitgeber is presented.

Polysomnogram   The sleep recording that displays brain activity, eye movement, and motor activity. Used by sleep researchers as a diagnostic and clinical tool.

REM sleep   Sleep characterized by rapid eye movement, brain activity close to that of wakefulness, and a complete absence of muscle tone. Most dreaming takes place during REM sleep.

REM Sleep Behavior Disorder (RBD)   A disorder marked by the loss of the normal paralysis that accompanies REM sleep, marked by complex and often violent behavior that occurs while the sleeper is in REM sleep.

Seasonal Affective Disorder (SAD)   A form of clinical depression in which a person becomes depressed every year during certain months—particularly during the fall and winter, when day lengths are shorter.

Sleep cycle   The approximately 90- to 100-minute cyclic fluctuations containing both REM and NREM sleep.

Sleep deprivation   Term used to describe the state you're in when you don't obtain enough sleep to satisfy the needs of your body and mind. Symptoms—the severity of which depend on both how sleep deprived you are and how sensitive your body is to the loss of sleep—may include daytime sleepiness, fatigue, irritability and mood swings, itchy eyes, fatigue, appetite changes, inability to concentrate, and others.

Sleep hygiene   Those practices of daily living that promote good sleep, including eating a proper diet, getting regular exercise, creating a conducive sleep environment, and others.

Sleep inertia   The symptoms of confusion and grogginess that may occur upon awakening, especially from deep Stages 3 and 4 of sleep.

Sleep paralysis   A brief episode of partial or total paralysis occurring at the beginning or end of a sleep period, usually occurring to people with narcolepsy.

Sleepwalking   A parasomnia that involves a sleeping person who leaves the bed and walks around in or outside of the house. Also called somnambulism.

Snoring   The hoarse sound of breathing during sleep that occurs when the soft palate vibrates. Excessive snoring may indicate Obstructive Sleep Apnea, a serious and common sleep disorder.

Sudden Infant Death Syndrome   The sudden death of an infant, during sleep, with no known cause; the leading cause of death in infants between the first month and first year of life.

Sundown syndrome   The recurrent appearance of behavioral disturbances such as agitation, aggression, pacing and restlessness during the late afternoon or evening among elderly or demented patients.

Suprachiasmatic nucleus of the hypothalamus (SCN)   A tiny cluster of brain cells that serve as the body's primary circadian biological clock, helping to orchestrate the sleep/wake cycle and a host of other physiological functions.

Teeth grinding   The grinding of teeth during sleep caused by tension, or a malalignment of the teeth within the jaw. Also called bruxism.

Tryptophan   One of the essential amino acids found in a variety of foods that is the precursor to serotonin, a known sleep promoter.

Ultradian rhythms   Biological rhythms that recur during a period shorter than 24 hours, such as the REM/NREM cycle of sleep that recurs every 90 to 100 minutes during the night.

Uvulopalatopharyngoplasty (UPPP)   Surgery used to correct Obstructive Sleep Apnea. It involves the trimming of excess tissue of the soft palate and other tissue to reconstruct the air space, allowing clear breathing during the sleep.

Zeitgeber   From the German meaning "time giver," an environmental cue (particularly light) that helps entrain the body's rhythm to the 24-hour day.

Index